بِسْمِ اللَّهِ الرَّحْمَنِ الرَّحِيم

SECOND EDITION

Print ISBN 978-1-7775152-3-2
eBook ISBN 978-1-7775152-6-3

www.dryoumethod.com
Instagram: @dr.you.official

TABLE OF CONTENTS

» What is this book?

This book is a compilation of some of the highest-yield and most memorable mnemonics in anatomy, as well as important (and often normally confusing) concepts and facts that I have made intuitive and easy to understand. It comprises mnemonics created by myself, as well as those learned from various sources during my studies.

It is designed to provide the most benefit in the least amount of time. As such, effort was made to concisely deliver the necessary points while avoiding unnecessary details.

The content is geared towards anatomy as taught in medical school and as tested on medical board examinations like the USMLE step 1 and step 2 CK. The content is especially useful for students learning introductory anatomy in first year, nonetheless much of it is likely to be encountered and tested on again in upper years due to its clinical significance.

Consideration was given to long-term memorability - in other words, I made an effort to include mnemonics that have stood the test of time and proven fruitful years later in my experience.

Have a great time reading and be sure to follow me on Instagram for new content on going above and beyond in medical school! I also create plans for getting you through (and acing) medical school, so visit: dryoumethod.com/ineedhelp

Dr. You

Instagram: @dr.you.official
www.dryoumethod.com

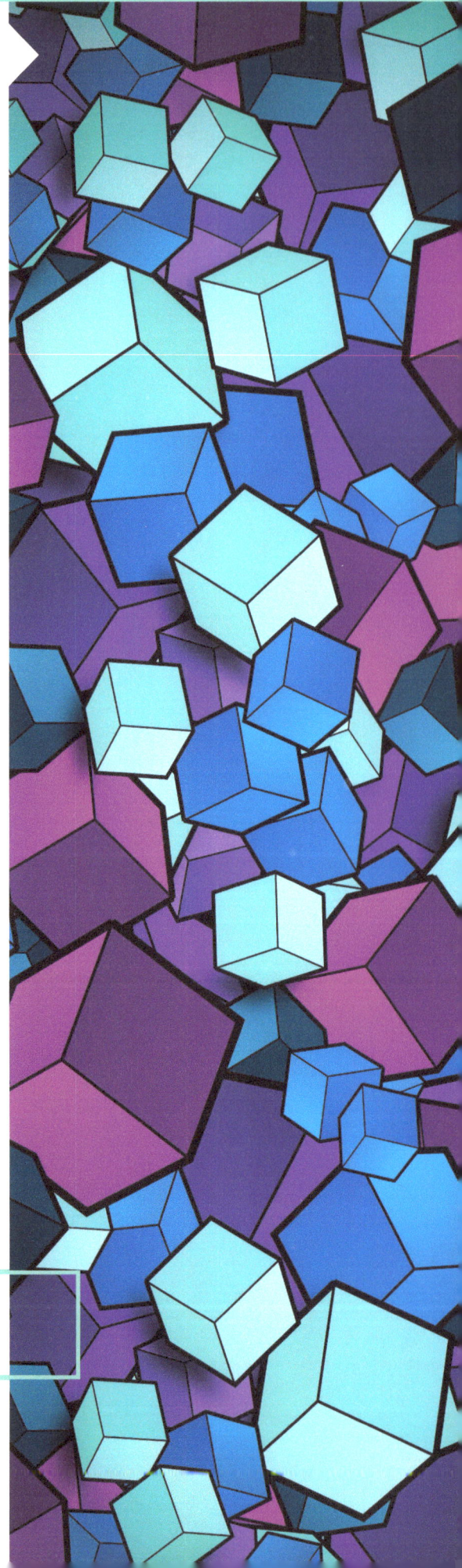

How to use this book

It is recommended to use one or both of the following approaches:

>> APPROACH #1 (preferred): Pre-reading + review

When beginning to study a particular organ system (e.g. musculoskeletal), read all of the mnemonics for that system **beforehand**. Then review them again after 1-2 days to ensure you understand and remember them. You can then proceed to learn the system in detail, having a mental map of all of the mnemonics within it. Then whenever needed, return to the mnemonics that require reviewing.

>> APPROACH #2: Search as needed

When encountering difficulty learning particular facts using traditional methods, check the appropriate chapter in this book or search the table of contents to see if there is a mnemonic for it. If using the eBook version, simply search using *Ctrl + F* (PC) or clicking on 🔍 in Kindle. Using this method exclusively is not recommended unless the subject has already been learnt thoroughly and all that is needed is a bit of extra review.

<u>The color red</u>
Whenever you see words highlighted in **red**, it signifies that the mnemonic or memory aid lies within those words. For example: "**T10** innervates the belly **butTEN**".

≫ A Quick Word on Mnemonics

Long "phrase" mnemonics that use the first letter of each word in the phrase to help you remember a series of medical words should be ***avoided*** unless truly necessary. There are a few exceptions – namely for certain anatomical parts that are particularly numerous, confusing, and difficult to remember. In such cases they may be quite beneficial if used correctly. You may see a select few examples of such mnemonics in this book.

As a general rule however, try to steer clear of these types of mnemonics. Although they may provide some short term benefit, they tend to perform very poorly in respect to **long-term memory**. An example of such a mnemonic is:

<u>M</u>y <u>V</u>ery <u>E</u>xcited <u>M</u>other <u>J</u>ust <u>S</u>erved <u>U</u>s <u>N</u>oodles =
<u>M</u>ercury, <u>V</u>enus, <u>E</u>arth, <u>M</u>ars, <u>J</u>upiter, <u>S</u>aturn, <u>U</u>ranus, <u>N</u>eptune

To retrieve the information from this mnemonic, you have to remember all the parts of the mnemonic, including what the mnemonic was for exactly and what each word represents. A crack in any layer of information means the mnemonic becomes of little value (which inevitably happens after some time). You may end up spending more time trying to remember what "mother just served us" than about understanding medicine. In medicine, the ability to mentally navigate in and out of concepts fluidly is of particular importance. For this reason, this book's emphasis is on intuitive and memorable mnemonics.

CHAPTER 1

Approach to Anatomy

CHAPTER 1: Approach to anatomy

Below are simple steps to make your anatomy studying significantly more efficient. However their principles are applicable to your medical education as a whole, and may help you in your academic life for years to come. Hang onto them!

⟫ No way around repetition

Mnemonics or no mnemonics - when it comes to learning anatomy there is no way around repetition. Using effective techniques can make your learning significantly easier and decrease the amount of time you have to spend in review, however you still need to solidify that memory by seeing the material more than once. This is a reliable principle to fall back on when learning even the most confusing anatomical facts and concepts. Repeat, repeat, repeat. Draw it out. List things out. Approach it differently. This is especially important when you've identified an area of weakness.

⟫ Spaced repetition

A big mistake many students make is to think all repetition is equal. It's *NOT*, and it might be wasting large amounts of your time. Repetition to solidify your memory of something is most effectively done in **increasingly-spaced intervals**. There are key points where we forget a newly learned fact, & recalling/reviewing the information at those points can allow for consolidating your long-term memory of it in the least amount of review time.

Review an anatomical fact a dozen times over within 2 days & you'll still likely forget it by 2 weeks. But with strategically-timed recall, 3 reviews might last you months or even years.

In my experience, the optimal intervals for recollection and review of material for anatomy is roughly:

1. Learn the material

2. Recall/review ~10 minutes later

(2.5. Optional: recall/think about it while you're in bed)

3. Recall/review the next day

4. Look over it before the midterm exam

5. Look over it before the final exam

Recall over recognition

Don't mistake recognition with recall. Recall - being able to mentally reconstruct the anatomical part on your own - is better than simply being able to recognize it. Recognition has a tendency to hit roadblocks when the exam presents the information with a slight variation. Recall entails a more thorough level of understanding.

Therefore when reviewing for an exam, avoid going straight to your notes and looking at the information. Instead, see if you can recreate the anatomical part on your own, either in your head or on paper. That not only strengthens your memory and understanding of it, but will identify where the gaps in your understanding lie.

Draw it out

One of your most effective tools for consolidating your understanding of a given anatomical region is drawing it out. As mentioned previously, doing so forces you to bring to your attention the gaps in your memory and understanding. It also solidifies your memory in ways that mental revision alone may not. Keep your drawings extremely simple though. You don't have unlimited time, so avoid unnecessary detail and effort making it look pretty.

≫ Study each region systematically

Anatomy comes with an intimidating number of facts and bits of information. To ensure you cover the most important parts of each body region as well as to simplify your studying, approach each region systematically. There are a number of ways to do this. For example, you can approach each limb using a set template covering all of the major structures:

1. Bones:
2. Muscles:
3. Arteries:
4. Veins:
5. Nerves:
6. Lymphatics:

≫ Group information into compartments

Retaining the immense amount of information in anatomy can be difficult if it is scattered chaotically in your brain. Our minds find it much easier to remember information when it is grouped into nice little compartments. So wherever possible, categorize the information. For example, there are 11 main muscles in the thigh. Instead of remembering the functions, blood supply, and innervation of each of these, they can be remembered in 3 simple compartments, each of which all have the same general functions, blood supply, and innervation.

» Number things

When presented with a set of related anatomical facts that you need to memorize, number them. Doing so can improve your recall of those items significantly. Try memorizing, for example, the branches of the external carotid artery: superior thyroid, ascending pharyngeal, lingual, facial, occipital, posterior auricular, maxillary, superficial temporal.

Now try memorizing them after numbering them. The **8** branches are:

1. Superior thyroid
2. Ascending pharyngeal
3. Lingual
4. Facial
5. Occipital
6. Posterior auricular
7. Maxillary
8. Superficial temporal

Notice any difference?

» Think about the name

Pay very close attention to the names of things - often the name will tell you critical (and memorable) information about it, and make remembering it (especially when you have thousands of other things to remember) significantly easier.

For example, the names of most of the rotator cuff muscles tell you about their relative locations. The name **"supraspinatus"** tells you the muscle lies **above** the scapular **spine**, while **"infraspinatus"** tells you it lies **below** it. From their locations, you can also determine their functions (provided you know their general area of insertion) by simply imagining what happens when you pull on the muscle. Knowing that all 4 rotator cuffs insert roughly around the lateral edge of the humerus, you can understand why the supraspinatus abducts the arm (as it comes from above) and the infraspinatus laterally rotates it. All of this information is retrieved by simply thinking about the name.

≫ First look at the forest, *then* the trees

Many topics in medicine can be overwhelming when attempting to learn them in detail all at once. This is especially the case with anatomy, where the sheer amount of detail can often make it difficult to come out remembering anything at all. It is therefore important to study each concept or body region in layers - beginning with an extremely simplified version and subsequently going over it in increasingly greater detail. Doing so allows you to solidify a clear and simple mental image of the concept upon which you can later build on. Without this clear mental image, a mere collection of scattered facts is likely all that you will retain, making subsequent studying of it disordered and confusing.

For example, when learning the branches of the abdominal aorta, instead of trying to learn the major branches and each of their runoff branches all at once, along with the organs they supply, a good first run-through would look like this:

There are <u>three</u> major branches of the abdominal aorta:

1. Celiac trunk (top one; supplies "foregut")
2. Superior mesenteric artery (middle one; supplies "midgut")
3. Inferior mesenteric artery (lowest one; supplies "hindgut")

That's it! Nice and simple. In a subsequent run-through you can then add on details like the branches of each major branch, etc.

For the same reason, it is also important to begin learning a body region from simplistic images that contain minimal levels of detail. You need to clearly see the forest before you start looking at all the trees!

≫ Be willing to change everything

If a particular resource or strategy isn't working for you, change it immediately. Some have a tendency to cling onto their old methods because it worked for them in the past. However you don't have unlimited time to "figure things out", so persisting with something that isn't working can prove disastrous.

If your textbook isn't working for you, turn to Google Images or YouTube videos. If attending lectures aren't proving too fruitful, study on your own. If your memorization techniques are too slow, let them go. The point is, be ready and willing to change as soon as you feel it might be advantageous.

≫ Resources

Your course PowerPoint slides are generally necessary to answer questions on your school exams, but they tend to be a fairly mediocre resource for actually learning anatomy. To accelerate the process of your actual learning and understanding of anatomy, it would be wise to supplement your slides with additional resources.

In my opinion, two of the most invaluable resources for learning anatomy (in addition to this book, of course!) are YouTube videos and Google Images. With most resources, you're fairly limited in terms of the content you get. In the case of YouTube, you have an immense number of content creators producing videos, and typically the best and most effective videos get the most views. You are therefore often able to find some of the most well-taught anatomy explanations with a simple search. In the case of Google Images, you generally have the ability to find images of a given body part with an immense variation of perspectives and levels of detail. Be sure to cross-check for accuracy if viewing images from less prominent sources though.

CHAPTER 2

General Principles & Terminology

1 Spatial terminology master page

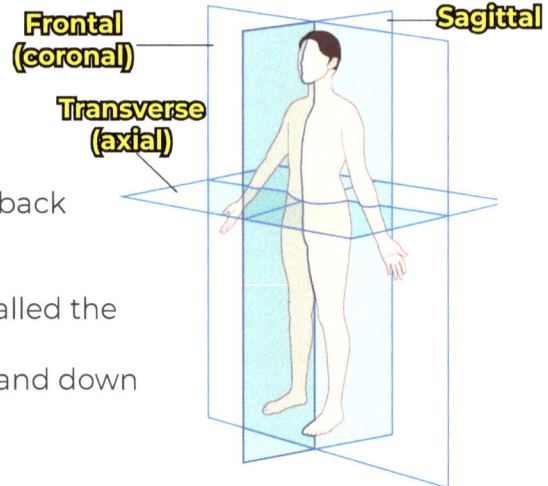

Frontal (coronal)
Sagittal
Transverse (axial)

The 3 planes

Since we live in 3 dimensions, there are 3 planes:

Frontal (coronal) plane: divides the body into front and back
Sagittal: divides the body vertically into right and left
- A big belly *sags* along the *sagittal* plane
- The sagittal plane that's exactly in the **mid**line is called the **midsagittal** or **median plane**

Transverse (axial): divides the body horizontally into up and down
- Think about how you *ax* a tree

Directional terms

Anterior vs. posterior: at the front (*anterior*) vs. at the back (*posterior*)
Superior vs. inferior: above (*superior*) vs. below (*inferior*)
Superficial vs. deep: closer to surface (*superficial*) vs. deeper into body (*deep*)
Proximal vs. distal: closer to trunk (*proximal*) vs. further out from it (*distal*)
Medial vs. lateral: closer to midline (*medial*) vs. further (*lateral*)

Less common:
Cranial vs. caudal: towards cranium i.e. top of head (*cranial*) vs. towards feet (*caudal*)
Ventral vs. dorsal: front (*ventral*) vs. back (*dorsal*) of an <u>embryo</u> before limb rotation
- Think of the *dorsal fin* of a fish.

Movements

Flexion vs. extension: decreasing the angle between the body parts (*flexion*) vs. increasing it (*extension*)

Abduction vs. adduction: pulling a body part away from the midline (*abduction*) vs. towards it (*adduction*)
- *adduction is adding the part to you*

Internal (medial) vs. external (lateral) rotation: rotation towards (*internal*) vs. away from (*external*) body's center

Elevation vs. depression: movement in the superior (*elevation*) vs. inferior (*depression*) direction

Special hand/feet movements

Dorsiflexion vs. plantarflexion: flexing the foot up (dorsiflexion) vs. extending it down (plantarflexion)
- *Think: planting your foot down*

Pronation vs. supination: rotating the forearm so the palm faces down (pronation) vs. up (supination)
- *Think: holding a bowl of soup*

Inversion vs. eversion: turning the sole of the foot towards midline (inversion) vs. away from it (eversion)

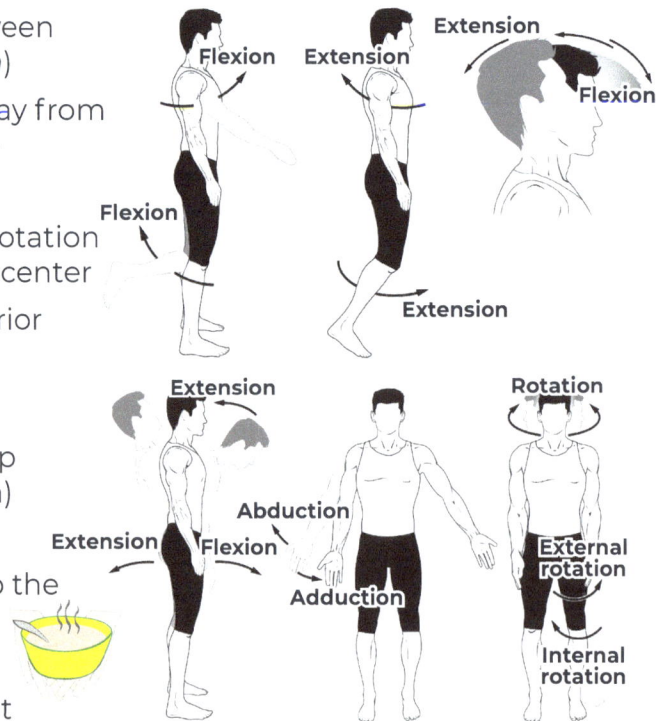

Flexion Extension
Extension
Flexion
Flexion
Extension

Extension
Abduction
Adduction
Extension Flexion

Rotation
External rotation
Internal rotation

2 Muscle terminology

Attachments

- **Origin:** the end that is **closest** to your core
- **Insertion:** the end that is **furthest** from your core

A muscle pulls the body part towards the muscle **origin**.

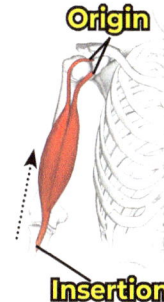

Naming

Some muscles are named according to their characteristics, like their size or shape. Knowing the meanings of these names can help you visually recognize them, understand their functions, and more.

By size

- **Longus vs. brevis:** In a pair of muscles, *longus* refers to the *longer* muscle and *brevis* to the *briefer* (i.e. shorter).
  - e.g. *peroneus longus* and *brevis*
- **Maximus/major vs. minimus/minor:** In a pair of muscles, *maximus* or *major* refers to the *larger* muscle and *minor* or *minimus* to the *smaller*.
  - e.g. *gluteus maximus* and *minimus*, *teres major* and *minor*, *pectoralis major* and *minor*

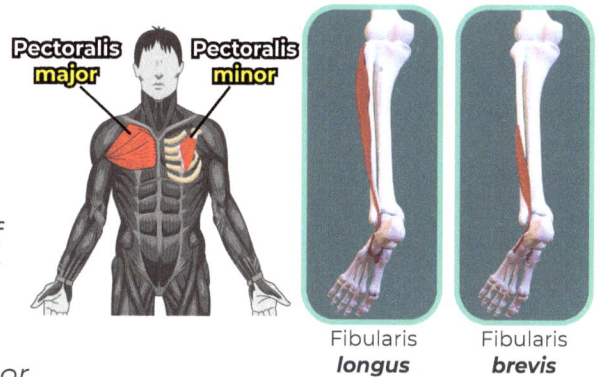

Fibularis *longus*

Fibularis *brevis*

By shape

- **Quad**ratus: Having *four* sides
  - e.g. *pronator quadratus*
- **Rhomboid:** Shaped like a *rhombus*
- e.g. *rhomboid major* and *minor*
- **Teres:** *round*
  - Like when you try to *tear* off a square of toilet paper but end up with a *rounded* edge
  - e.g. *teres major* and *minor*; also applies to non-muscle things too, like *ligamentum teres* (round ligament of the liver)
- **Bi**ceps/**tri**ceps/**quad**riceps: Simply mean the muscle has *two, three,* or *four* parts, respectively.
  - e.g. *biceps brachii, biceps femoris, triceps, quadriceps*

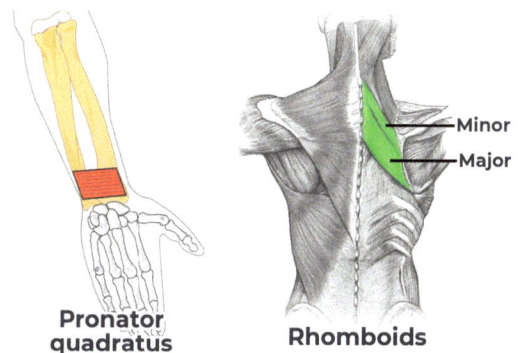

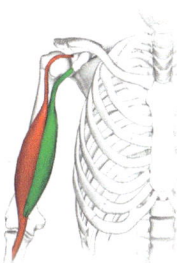

Pronator quadratus

Rhomboids

Minor

Major

Biceps brachii

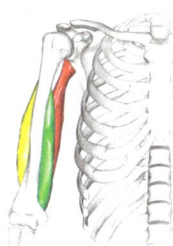

Triceps

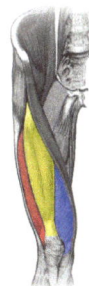

Quadriceps
(the 4th part, the vastus intermedius, is deep and not seen)

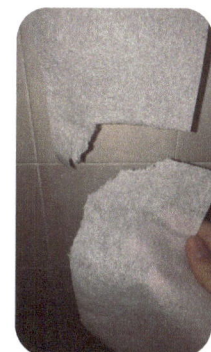

Paperus teres - extremely common variant of the *paperus quadratus*

3   Parietal vs. visceral

> The **Parietal** layer is the **Parent** (covering and protecting the visceral layer).

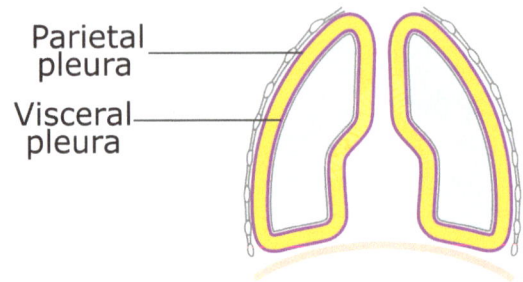

Parietal pleura

Visceral pleura

When referring to the linings of an organ:
- **Parietal** is the _outer layer_;
- **Visceral** is the _inner_ (organ-lining) _layer_.

The pair of terms "parietal" and "visceral" is seen in 3 main areas:

1. **Heart (pericardium)**
2. **Lungs (pleura)**
3. **Abdominal cavity (peritoneum)**.

On occasion, you might see one of the terms outside of this context. Internal organs are sometimes called _"viscera"_, and the brain has a _parietal lobe_.

(!) **Accumulations between parietal and visceral layers:** Problems can arise when a substance accumulates between the parietal and visceral layers of the pericardium and pleura (normally EMPTY). In the lung, a break in the pleura can pump air into the pleural space like a balloon, compressing the lung - called a **pneumothorax**. In the heart, blood can accumulate in the pericardial space - called a **hemopericardium**. It can compress the heart so much that it leads to insufficient blood outflow (called **cardiac tamponade**) and death! The abdominal cavity is huge, so acute compression emergencies (called **abdominal compartment syndrome**) are less common and mainly happen in patients who are already critically ill.

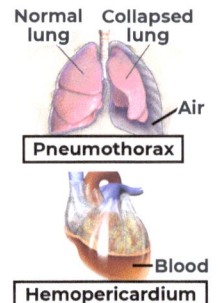

Normal lung   Collapsed lung
Air
Pneumothorax

Blood
Hemopericardium

4   Cortex vs. medulla

- **Cortex:** the **ex**terior part of an organ
- **Medulla:** the interior part of an organ (the _"middle"_)

Cortex

Medulla

The major organs that contain the pair of terms are:

1. kidneys
2. adrenal glands
3. thymus
4. brain

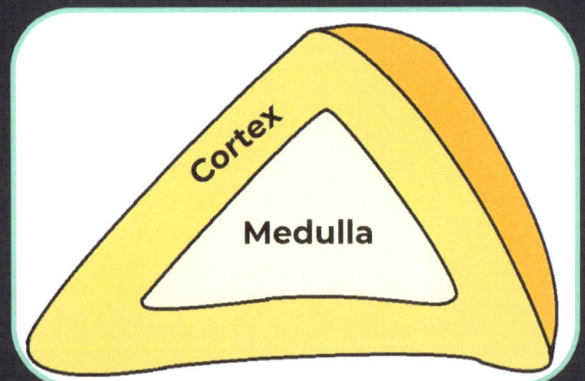

Dr.You
METHOD

5 Fundus

> **The fundus of an organ is the part that is *furdus* (furthest) from the opening.**

The **major fundi** of the body are located in the:

1. Urinary bladder

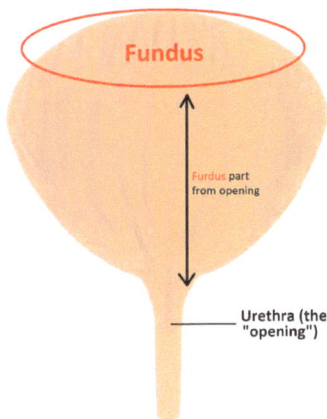

Fundus

Furdus part from opening

Urethra (the "opening")

2. Gallbladder

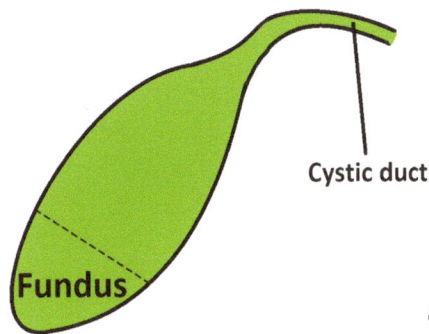

Cystic duct

Fundus

3. Stomach

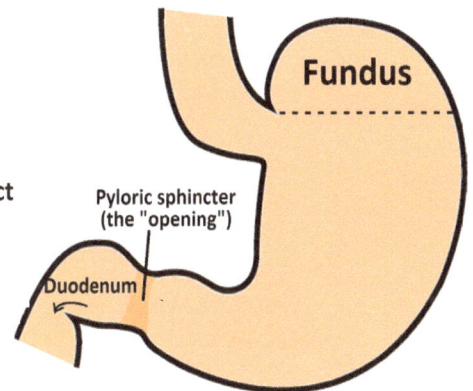

Fundus

Pyloric sphincter (the "opening")

Duodenum

4. Uterus

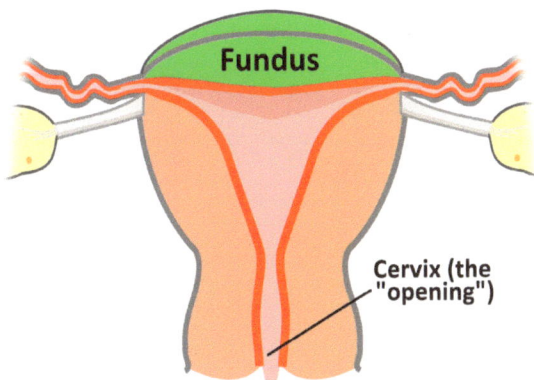

Fundus

Cervix (the "opening")

5. Eye

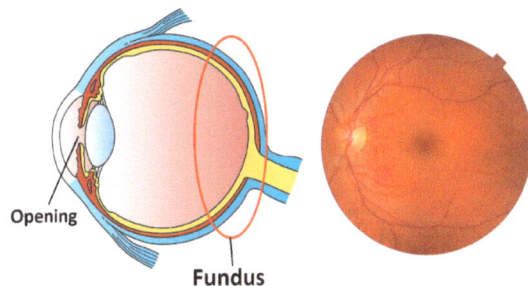

Opening

Fundus

View of the **fundus** using a **fundos**cope ("**fundos**copy")

6 Tubercle/tuberosity

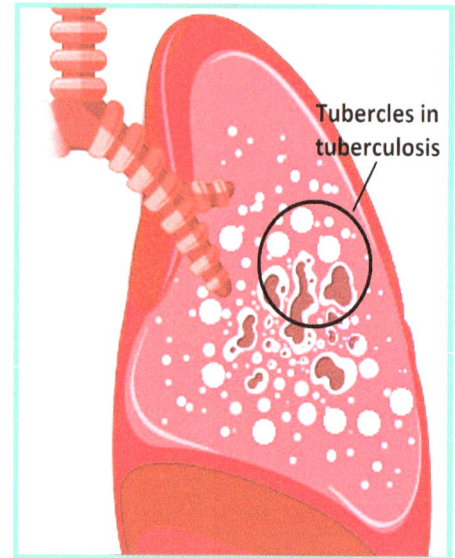

Tubercles in tuberculosis

Think of tuberculosis

A **tubercle** (also called a **tuber**osity) is a **small, rounded point of bone**. Remember this by thinking of the small, round balls of bacteria that **tubercul**osis (literally meaning **"a disease of tubercles"**) causes to form in your lungs.

Tubercles/tuberosities serve as **attachment sites for muscles**. The main tubercles of the body are located in the:

1. Humerus

Right Humerus

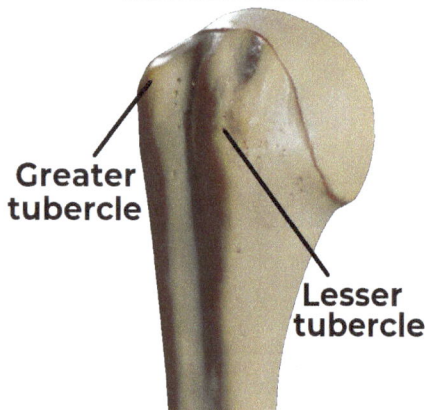

Greater tubercle

Lesser tubercle

2. Femur ("trochanter")

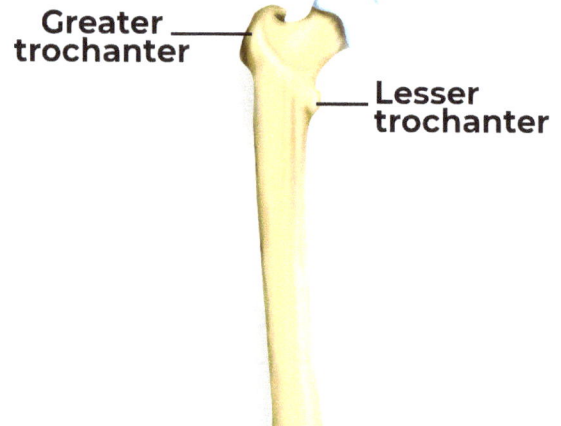

Greater trochanter

Lesser trochanter

3. Tibia (tuberosity)

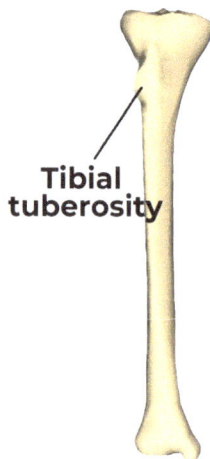

Tibial tuberosity

4. Ribs

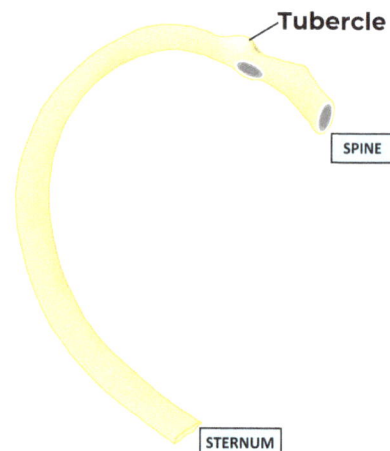

Tubercle

SPINE

STERNUM

14

7 Condyle and epicondyle

> **Condyle:** **knuckle**-like prominence at the end of a long bone.
> **Epicondyle:** the part that lies **upon** the **condyle**

A **condyle** (literally meaning **knuckle**) is the **round prominence** at the joint part of a long bone.
An **epicondyle** ('epi-' meaning **upon**) is the rounded eminence that lies upon the condyle.

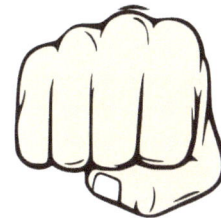

The **3 main sites of condyles** are:

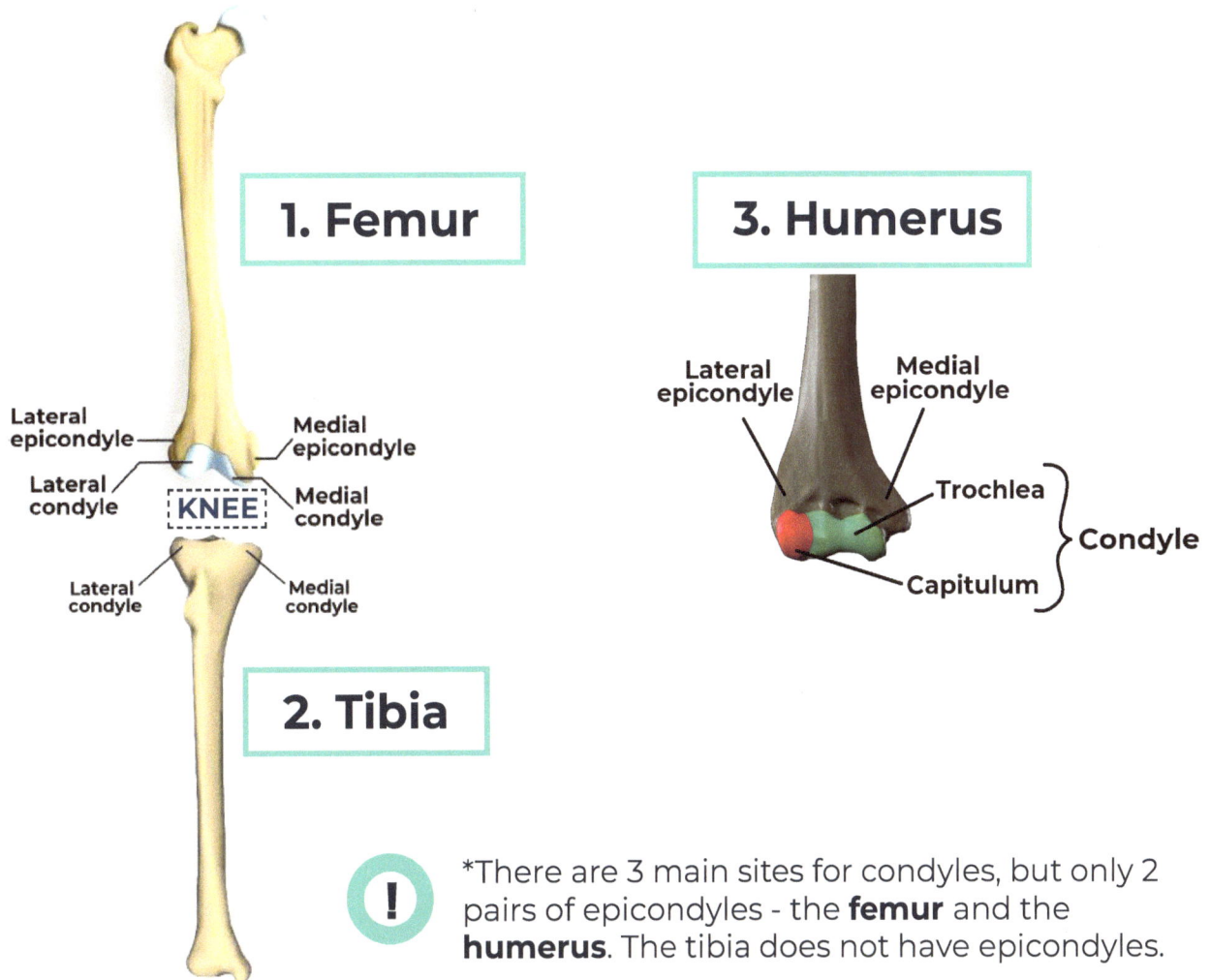

1. Femur

Lateral epicondyle
Medial epicondyle
Lateral condyle
KNEE
Medial condyle
Lateral condyle
Medial condyle

2. Tibia

3. Humerus

Lateral epicondyle
Medial epicondyle
Trochlea
} Condyle
Capitulum

! *There are 3 main sites for condyles, but only 2 pairs of epicondyles - the **femur** and the **humerus**. The tibia does not have epicondyles.

8   Fossa

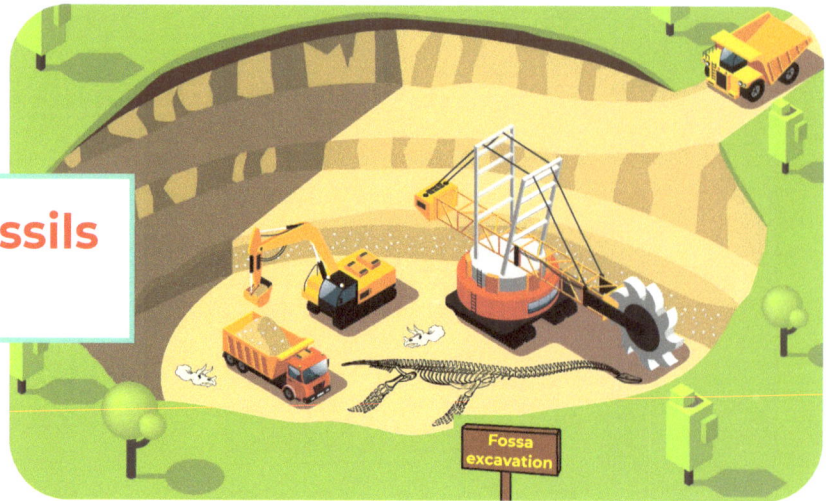

Think of digging for fossils beneath the ground.

A **fossa** is a **shallow depression or hollow**, usually in bone. Think of **fossil** dig sites, which likewise are depressions in the ground.

There are many fossae in the body, but very notable ones are:

The 3 cranial fossae

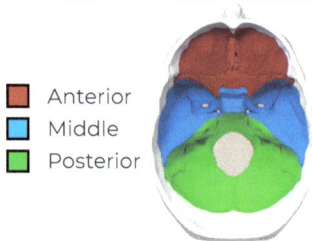

■ Anterior
■ Middle
■ Posterior

Iliac fossa

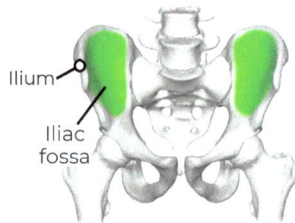

Ilium

Iliac fossa

Cubital fossa

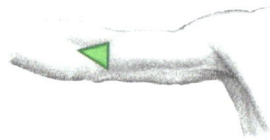

Fossa ovalis

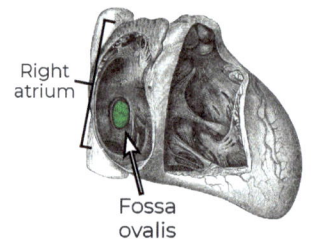

Right atrium

Fossa ovalis

9   Process

A process = a projection/ protrusion from a structure

A **process** is a very commonly used anatomical term meaning **projection** or **protrusion** from a structure. Remember that the prefix *'pro-'* means *advancing or projecting forward/outward*.

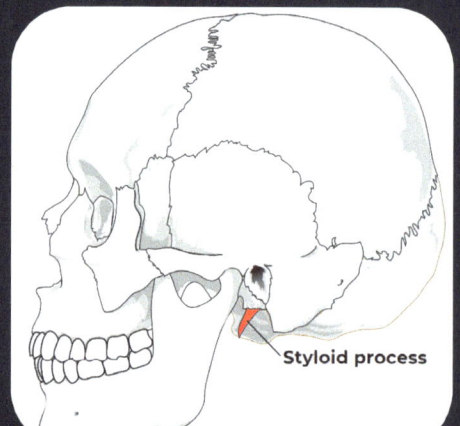

Styloid process

Styloid process (temporal)

(!) A **styloid process** is a process that resembles a **stylus (pen)** - hence narrow and pointy. The main styloid process to remember is the **temporal** styloid process *(see image)*. There's a radial and an ulnar styloid process at the wrist, but these are less commonly tested/discussed.

Other important processes include:

Mastoid process

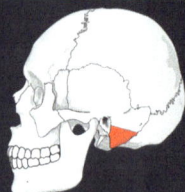

Xiphoid process

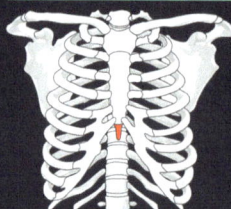

Acromion and coracoid processes (scapula)

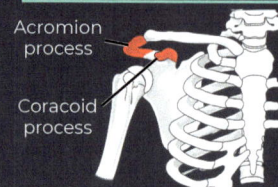

Acromion process

Coracoid process

10 Infundibulum

Infundibulum: a funnel-shaped cavity or structure

The major infundibula of the body are:

1. Pituitary gland

Also known as the "**pituitary stalk**", the pituitary infundibulum is the funnel-shaped connection between the hypothalamus and the posterior pituitary

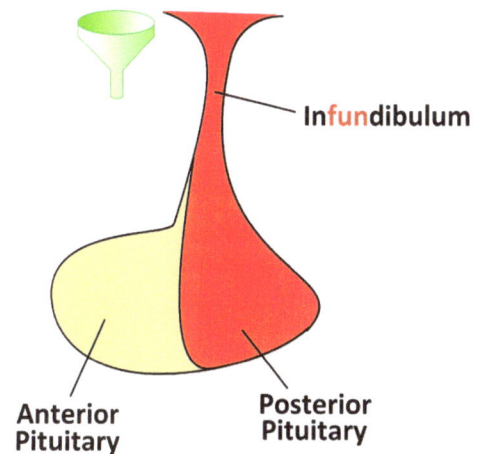

Infundibulum

Anterior Pituitary

Posterior Pituitary

2. Fallopian tube

The infundibulum of the fallopian tube is the funnel-shaped part closest to the ovary.

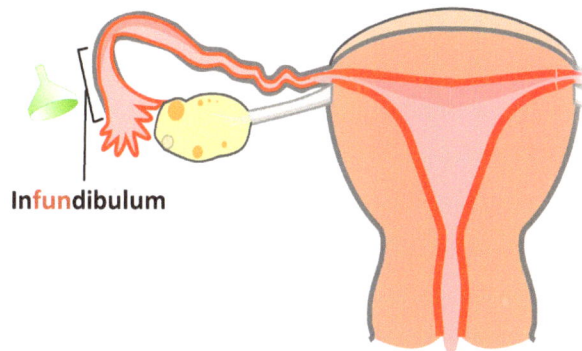

Infundibulum

3. Gallbladder

The infundibulum of the gallbladder, also called the **neck**, is the end closest to the cystic duct. It is a common site for gallstones to get stuck.

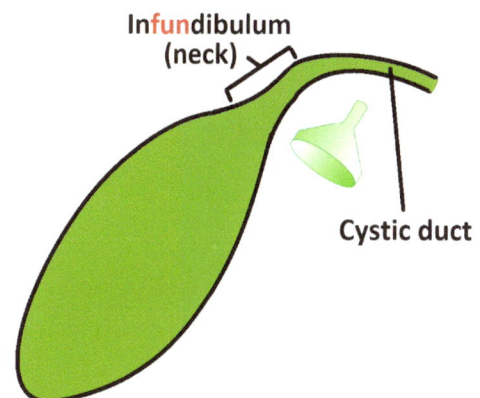

Infundibulum (neck)

Cystic duct

The renal pelvis is also occasionally called the *renal infundibulum.*

11   Fascia

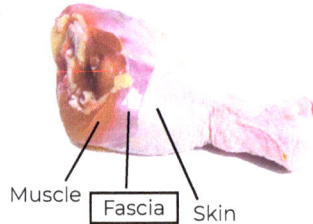

Copyright: Andrzej Pilat. Published with permission.

What is Fascia?

Fascia is a layer of **fibrous connective tissue** that surrounds muscles and internal organs. If you've ever handled raw chicken, it's that thin, shiny white-ish tissue that surrounds the muscles and keeps them whole.

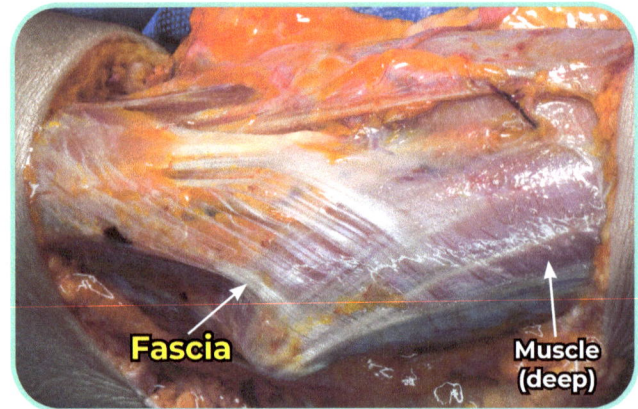

Muscle   Fascia   Skin

What does fascia do?

Fascia simply gives **structure** and **support** to muscles and organs, and also helps them stay neat and organized. Think of how a cord envelopes all the wires inside it.

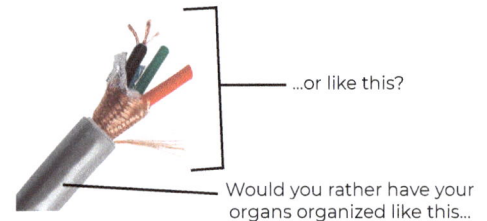

...or like this?

Would you rather have your organs organized like this...

Types of Fascia

You can categorize fascia into two groups: **muscle fascia** and **visceral fascia**.

1. Muscle ("deep") fascia

- Separates muscles into **compartments**
- Reduces friction with movement
- Protects the muscles' blood vessels and nerves from getting sheared with movement

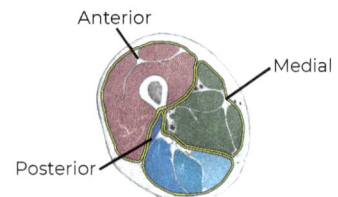

Anterior

Medial

Posterior

Thigh compartments

<u>Clinical significance</u>

Compartment syndrome: Since fascia encloses muscles of the upper and lower limbs into sealed compartments, significant swelling or internal bleeding into a compartment can **increase the pressure** in the compartment way too much. This high pressure can **squeeze off blood vessels** and cause the distal part of the limb to become ischemic and possibly die. The treatment is simply to cut the fascia of the compartment to release the pressure - this is called a **fasciotomy**!

2. Visceral fascia

- **Suspends** organs within their cavities
- Wraps organs in layers of connective tissue membranes
- E.g. Pericardium, pleura

<u>Clinical significance</u>

- **Adhesions:** Trauma (e.g. surgery) and inflammation (e.g. infections) can irritate fascia and cause it to become **sticky** and then eventually **fibrosed**. This can lead to organs sticking together in funny ways - these are called **adhesions**! Adhesions may cause problems like bowel obstruction or pain.

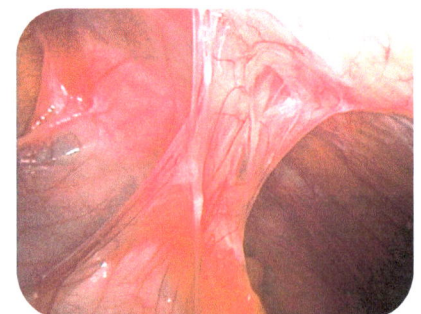

Abdominal adhesion after appendectomy

- **Organ prolapse:** If pelvic or abdominal fascia become too lax (e.g. after delivering twins), it can contribute to organ prolapse (rectal, uterine, bladder).

Dr. You
METHOD

12 Aponeurosis

Apple-neurosis

Aponeurosis: a **broad, flat, white tendon**

You know what else is broad, flat, and white? Exactly - an **Apple** iPad.
Alternatively, simply repeat the phrase "aponeurosis - a broad, flat tendon" several times (it's surprisingly catchy!)

As it's a tendon, aponeuroses connect **muscle to bone**. The major aponeuroses in the body are:

1. Plantar & palmar aponeuroses	2. Abdominal aponeurosis	3. Lumbar aponeurosis	4. Scalp aponeurosis

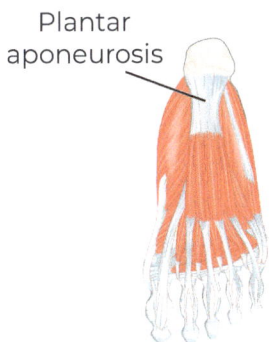

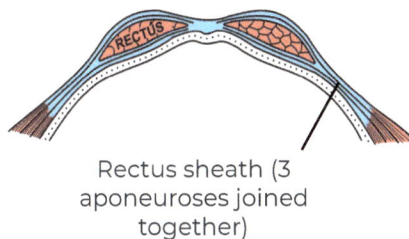

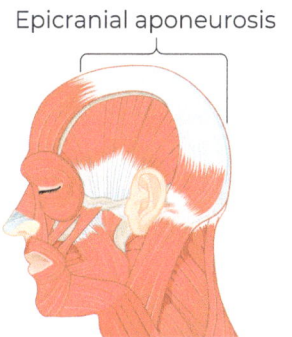

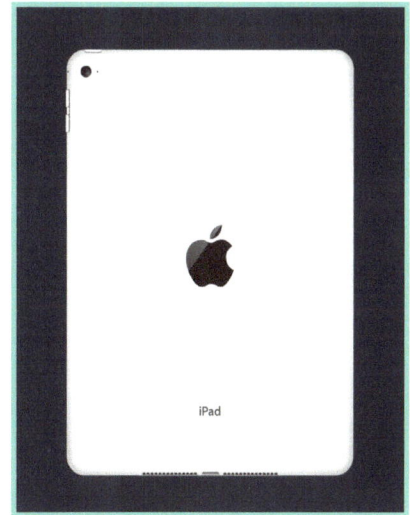

Plantar aponeurosis

Rectus sheath (3 aponeuroses joined together)

Thoracolumbar fascia (aponeurosis)

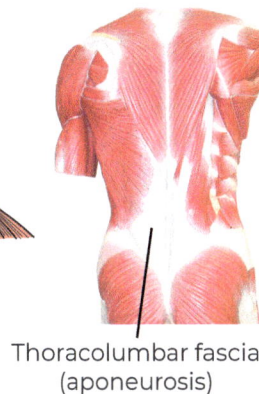

Epicranial aponeurosis

13 Foramen

Bore-amen

Foramen: an opening or hole through tissue, usually bone.

The word foramen literally means "**bore** a hole"!

A foramen allows blood vessels and nerves to pass from one side of the structure to the other. There are numerous foramina throughout the body - especially in the skull, for all those cranial nerves and vessels to pass through!

Remember - there are non-bony foramima too, including **foramen ovale** (heart) and the **epiploic foramen** (abdomen).

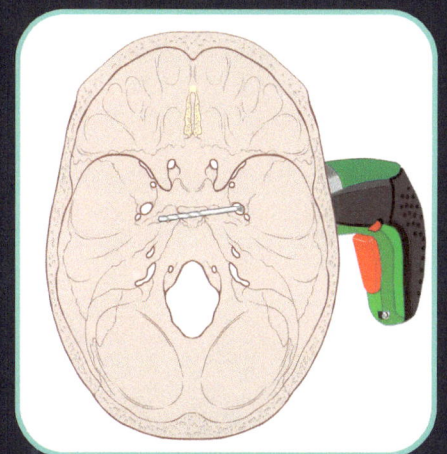

All of these holes are cranial foramina!

19

14 Miosis vs mydriasis

> **"Miosis: pupil closes"**
> **"'Mydri-': pupil wide"**

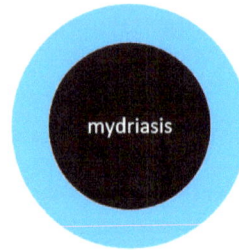

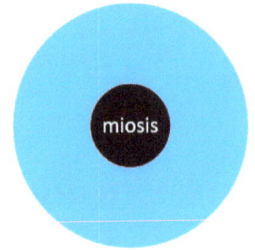

Miosis is the term for **constriction** of the pupil(s). It is facilitated by **parasympathetics** via **cranial nerve 3 (occulomotor nerve)**. Opioids are known to cause miosis.

Mydriasis is the term for **dilation** of the pupil(s). It is facilitated by **sympathetics**, and is often seen with use of a variety of drugs, including epinephrine, anti-cholinergics, amphetamines, and cocaine.

CHAPTER 3

General Musculoskeletal

15 Tendon vs. ligament

> **Tend**ons involve **tend**er tissues (muscles).

- **Tendon:** connects *bone* to *muscle*
- **Ligament:** connects *2 bones*

Alternative: Simply think of the **ligaments in your knee** (ACL, PCL, etc.) to remember that ligaments connect two bones together, or your **Achilles tendon** to remember tendons connect bones to muscle.

(!) **Tears:** Since ligaments stabilize joints, a tear to a ligament causes **joint instability**. On the other hand, since tendons anchor muscle to bone, a tear to a tendon causes **weakness**. A torn ligament can heal (albeit slowly) without surgery, but a completely ruptured tendon essentially never heals without surgery.

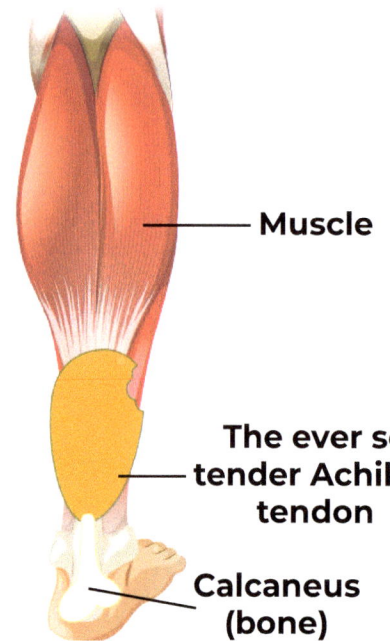

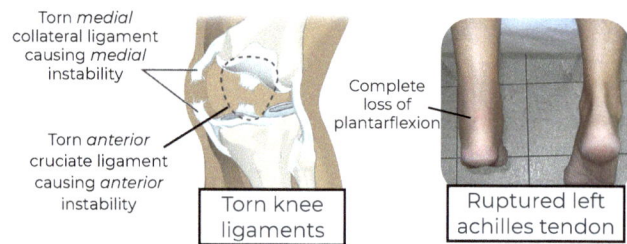

Muscle

The ever so tender Achilles tendon

Calcaneus (bone)

Torn *medial* collateral ligament causing *medial* instability

Complete loss of plantarflexion

Torn *anterior* cruciate ligament causing *anterior* instability

Torn knee ligaments

Ruptured left achilles tendon

16 Layers of the scalp

> **SCALP**

From superficial to deep:

Skin

Connective tissue

Aponeurosis (galea)

Loose connective tissue

Periosteum

An ideal mnemonic – where the mnemonic is literally the name of the thing you're trying to learn!

Danger zone: The **loose connective tissue** layer is known as the danger zone because **infections** can easily spread through it to the intracranial space via **emissary veins**.
Think: that's why they call it **loose**!

Dr.You
METHOD

17 Femoral triangle

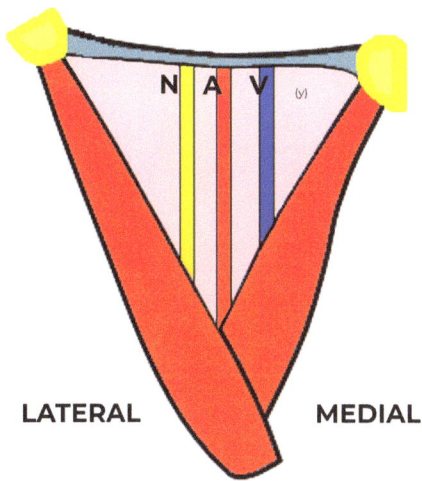

LATERAL   **MEDIAL**

a   Contents

NAVy

From lateral to medial:
- **N**erve (femoral nerve)
- **A**rtery (femoral artery)
- **V**ein (femoral vein)

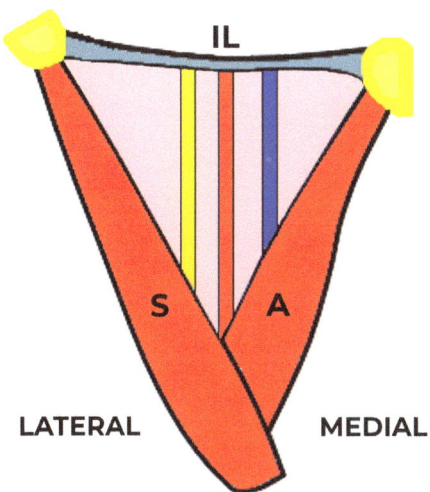

b   Borders

SAIL

- **S**artorius (lateral border)
- **A**dductor longus (medial border)
- **I**nguinal **L**igament (superior border)

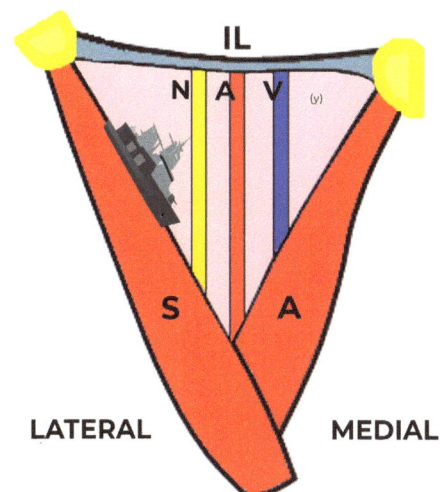

c   Contents + borders

The NAVy SAILs into the bermuda (femoral) TRIANGLE.

This is an immensely valuable (and rare) mnemonic in that it captures several layers of information in one short, intuitive phrase. Remember that the word "*into*" is used to denote that the contents are listed from **lateral to medial**. For added effect, vividly picture the scene in your mind.

18 Carotid sheath

> Inside the carotid sheath:
> **2 'internals', 2 'carotids',
> and the vagus nerve**

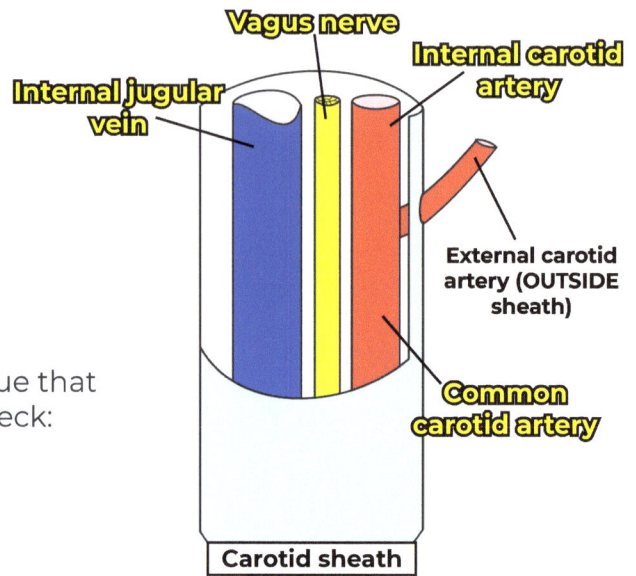

The carotid sheath is the sheath of connective tissue that bundles together the following structures in the neck:

1. Common **carotid** artery
2. **Internal carotid** artery
3. **Internal** jugular vein
4. Vagus nerve (CN 10)

- It makes sense that there are 2 'carotids' because this is the _carotid_ sheath after all...
- It makes sense that _INSIDE_ this sheath are the _'internal'_ branches of the two major neck vessels (carotid and jugular). The external branches obviously travel externally.

! The vein (jugular) is LATERAL to the artery (carotid) here. This is the _opposite_ of the femoral sheath/ triangle, where the vein is medial to the artery (remember "NAVy"?).

19 Neck triangles

> **Focus on the names + draw this square**

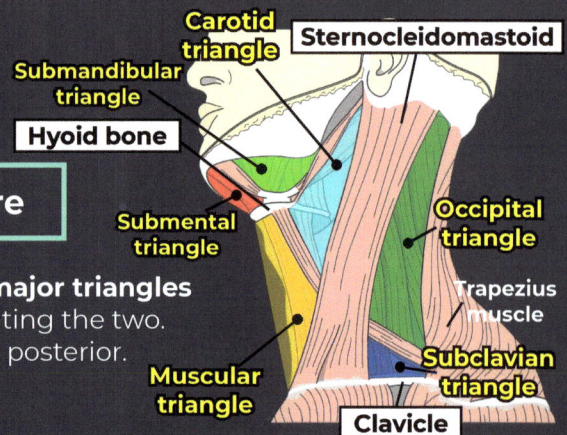

When viewed from the side, the neck can be divided into **two major triangles** - **anterior** and **posterior** - with the **sternocleidomastoid** separating the two. Within each are smaller triangles - **4** in the anterior and **2** in the posterior.

Anterior
1. Submental
2. Submandibular
3. Carotid
4. Muscular

Posterior
1. Occipital
2. Subclavian

Locations
The location of every triangle except the muscular triangle is found in its name.
- **Occipital**: by the **occiput** (back of head)
- **Subclavian**: right above the **clavicle** (even though it says 'sub-'...)
- **Submental**: **below** the **mentum** (chin)
- **Submandibular**: **below** the **mandible**
- **Carotid**: palpate your **carotid** artery on your own neck

Contents
Think about the location of each triangle to remember its contents.
- **Occipital**: accessory nerve (CN 11), cervical plexus
- **Subclavian**: **subclavian** artery
- **Submental**: lymph nodes
- **Submandibular**: parotid gland, lymph nodes, facial artery/vein
- **Carotid**: **carotid sheath** and its contents (see mnemonic)
- **Muscular**: thyroid & parathyroid glands, larynx, trachea, esophagus (all MIDLINE structures!)

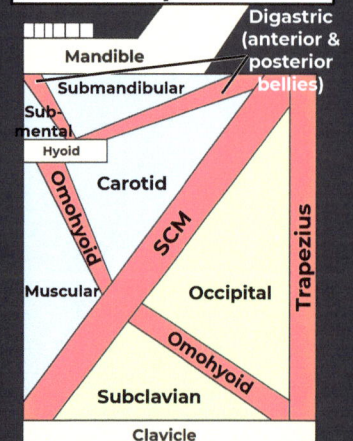

Practice drawing out this square a few times and it should make remembering the triangles and their borders significantly easier.

Dr.You
METHOD

20 Cubital fossa contents

TAN

From lateral to medial:
- **T**endon *(of biceps)*
- **A**rtery *(brachial)*
- **N**erve *(median)*

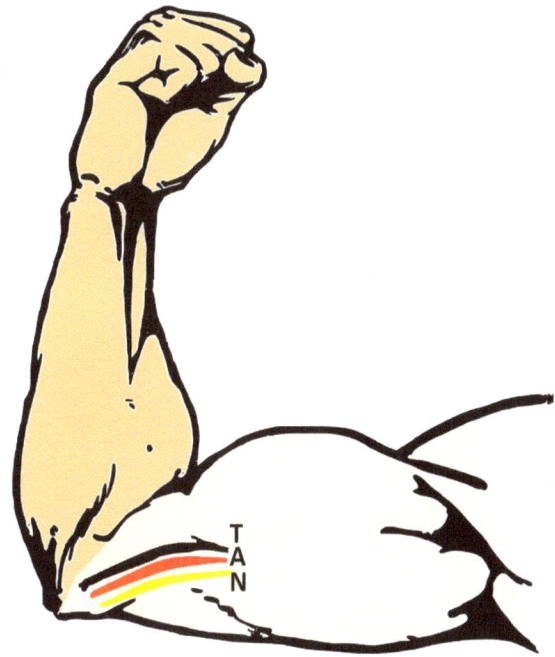

! You can remember that this mnemonic is referring to the **cubital fossa** because that's where you see a person's TAN line (if they've been wearing a t-shirt).

! An easy way to remember that the mnemonic goes from **lateral to medial** is to palpate your own arm and feel for your brachial pulse - you'll note that it's MEDIAL to your biceps tendon.

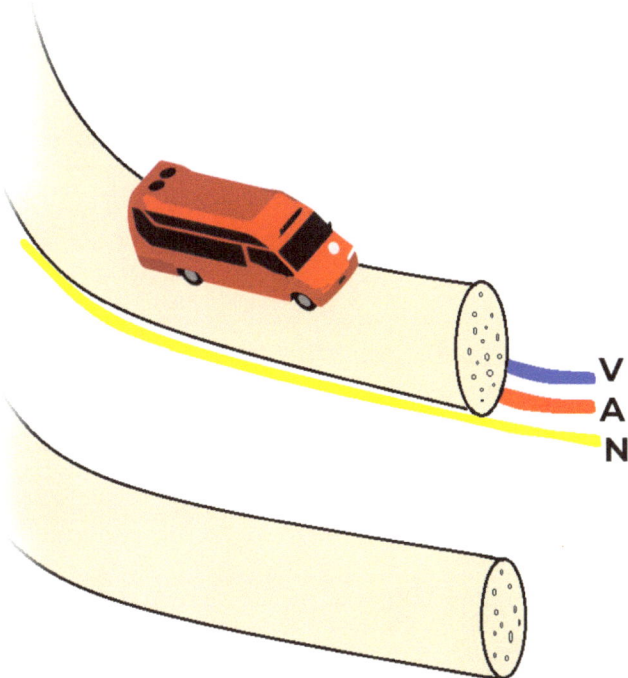

21 Intercostal vessels and nerves

VAN

From superior to inferior:
- **V**ein *(intercostal)*
- **A**rtery *(intercostal)*
- **N**erve *(intercostal)*

! You can remember that this mnemonic is referring to the **intercostal vessels/nerves** by imagining a **van** driving along the ribs (they look a bit like train tracks, don't they?)

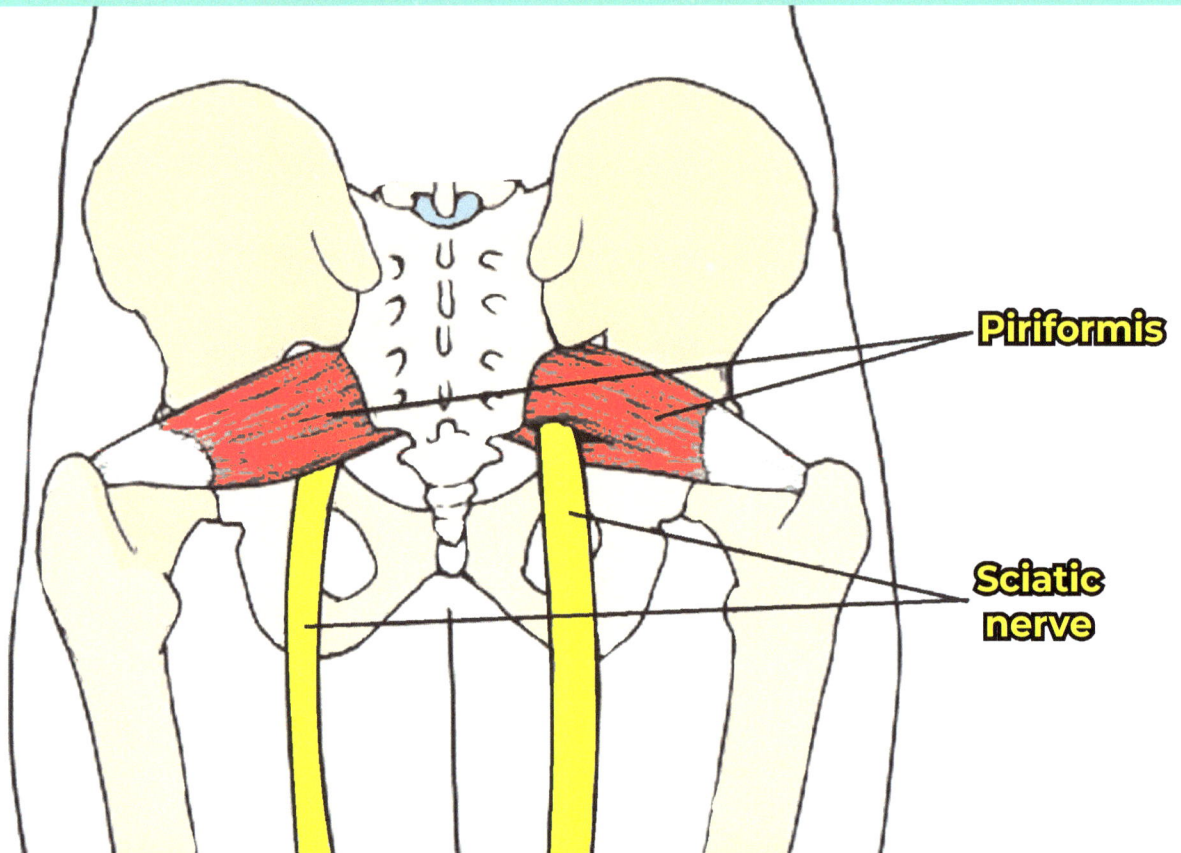

Piriformis

Sciatic nerve

22 Sciatic nerve emergence

The sciatic nerve perforates the piriformis

The piriformis serves as an excellent landmark for the sciatic nerve because of its unique appearance within that region. Find the piriformis and you'll find the sciatic nerve right there emerging from it.

The sciatic nerve originates from nerve roots **L4-S3**. It gives rise to the **tibial** and **common fibular (peroneal) nerves** just above the knee.

(!) **Piriformis syndrome:** Due to its location, the piriformis can irritate the sciatic nerve (e.g. chronically sitting on a fat wallet), causing *piriformis syndrome* - a type of **sciatica**. Pain, tingling, and numbness radiates down the back of the leg and into the foot (along the course of the sciatic nerve).

(!) **Straight leg raise test:** *Sciatica* is tested for via the *straight leg raise test*. With the patient lying flat on their back, the examiner raises their leg while keeping it straight. Pain radiating down the leg between **30-70°** suggests sciatic pain.

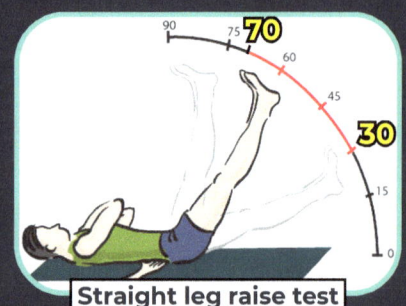

Straight leg raise test

SERRATOSAURUS ANTERIOR

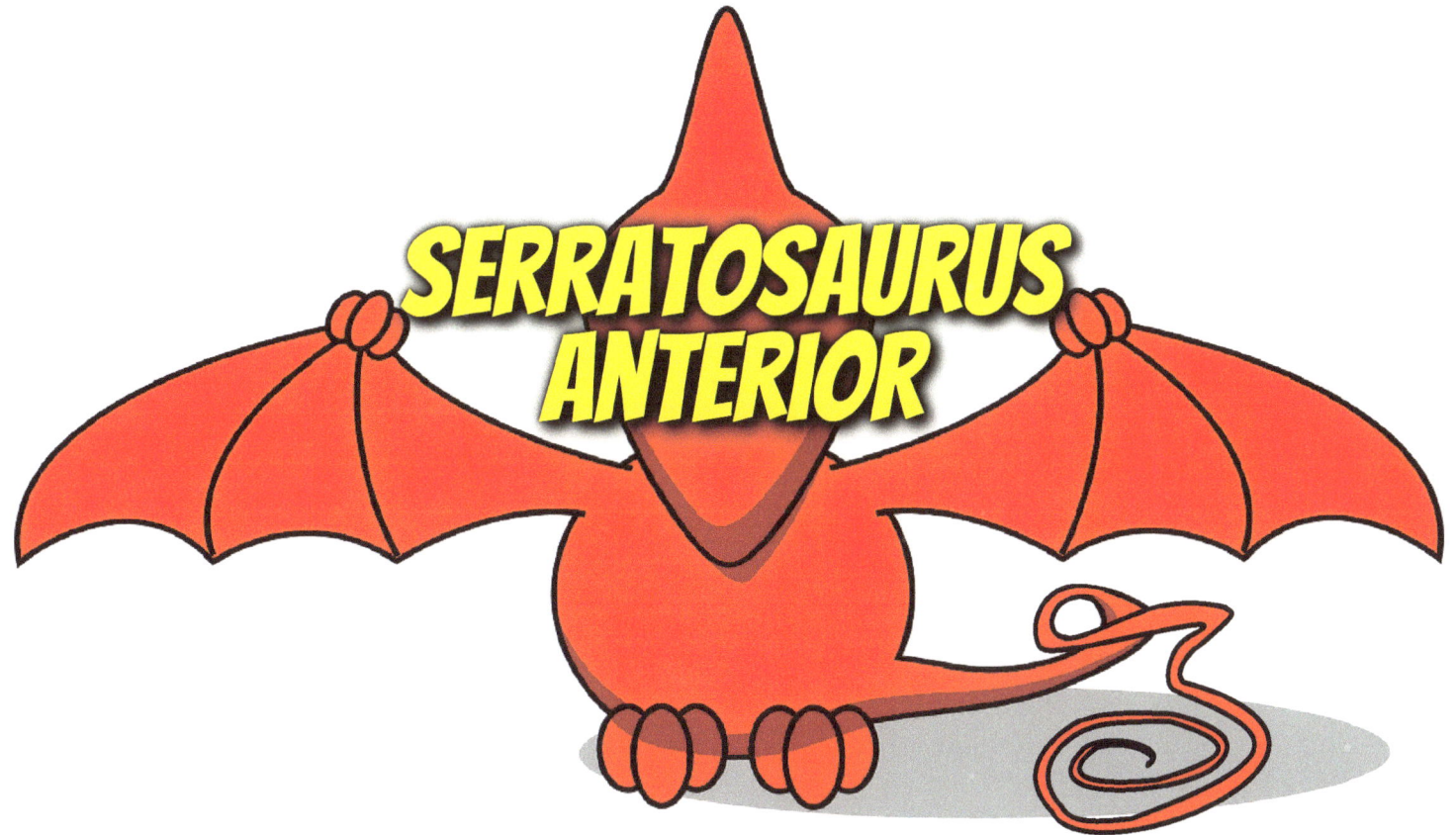

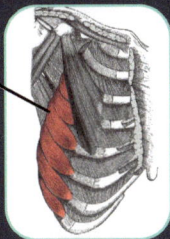

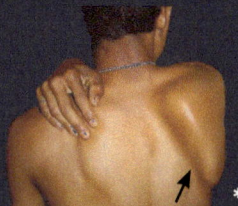

23 Serratus anterior

The serratus anterior muscle sounds an awful lot like a dinosaur, doesn't it?

Say hello to the fabled **serratosaurus anterior**! Its uncomfortably **long tail** should remind you of its innervation by the **long thoracic nerve**, and its widely-spread **wings** should remind you of the characteristic "**winged scapula**" deformity seen when the nerve is injured.

Think of the *Serratosaurus anterior*

Serratus anterior

Winged scapula

BONUS: Picture the serratosaurus as an avid boxer to remember that the serratus anterior is often called the "boxer's muscle" as it is largely responsible for protraction of the scapula (as happens during a punch).

NOTES

CHAPTER 4

Muscles, Tendons, & Ligaments

24 General rule: superficial vs. deep extremity muscles

> **Superficial muscle layers** are **bigger** and act on **bigger, proximal joints.**
> **Deep muscle layers** are **smaller** and act on **smaller, distal joints.**

The forearm, lower leg, and foot have different layers of muscles. A general principle to help remember them and their functions is that muscles in superficial layers tend to be bigger and act on bigger, proximal joints (in addition to more distal joints), while muscles in deeper layers tend to be smaller and act on smaller, distal joints.

To understand *why* this is true, it's important to visualize it. Take the gastrocnemius and soleus muscles of the calf, for example. The gastrocnemius is superficial and attaches ABOVE the knee - hence it can flex the knee. However its attachment site is **physically blocking the soleus from extending upward** above it because it's on top of it! Therefore, the soleus attaches BELOW the knee and does not flex it. Also, since the gastrocnemius essentially **encases** the soleus, it makes sense that the soleus (and deep muscles in general) is smaller than the gastrocnemius.

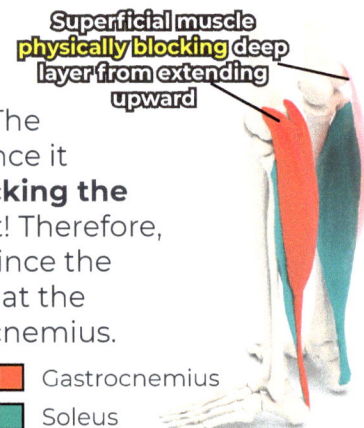

Superficial muscle physically blocking deep layer from extending upward

🟥 Gastrocnemius
🟩 Soleus

25 Anterior forearm muscles

$$4 = 1 + 3$$

In general, the anterior forearm muscles perform **flexion** (of wrist and fingers) and **pronation**.

There are **8** anterior forearm muscles, divided into 3 *levels* (or depths): **4 superificial, 1 intermediate**, and **3 deep** (remember the equation **4 = 1 + 3**):

- **Superficial** (4): **p**ronator teres, **f**lexor carpi radialis, **p**almaris longus, **f**lexor carpi ulnaris
  - From lateral to medial: *"pass, fail, pass, fail"*
- **Intermediate** (1): flexor digitorum superficialis
- **Deep** (3): flexor digitorum profundus, flexor policus longus, pronator quadratus

Memory tips:
- The superficial level is the only level that has *flexor **CARPI*** muscles (flexors of the wrist)! All deeper "flexors" are *finger* flexors (*digitorum* or *policis* ['policis' meaning 'thumb']).
- With the above in mind, the middle and deep layers are quite easy to remember: flexor digitorum SUPERFICIALIS would obviously be superficial to the flexor digitorum profundus – hence in the intermediate layer. The other two finger flexors are in the deep layer. The pronator quadratus is the odd one out.
- Remember: *'profundus'* means *deep*!

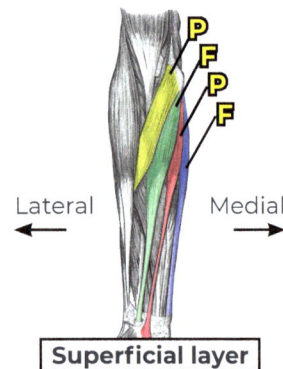

Lateral ← → Medial

Superficial layer

Innervation: All anterior forearm muscles are innervated by the **median nerve**, *EXCEPT* two that are innervated by the ulnar nerve: **1. flexor carpi *ulnaris*, 2. flexor digitorum *profundus*** ("*profoundly* different innervation").

❗ The **median nerve** and **ulnar artery** travel between the two heads of the **flexor digitorum superficialis** (intermediate layer), making the muscle a good landmark ("*the median nerve travels in the middle layer*").

26 Posterior forearm muscles

6 Superficial, 6 Deep

Known as the **extensor muscles**, the posterior forearm muscles generally perform **extension** (of wrist and fingers). There are **6 superficial** and **6 deep** muscles - separated by a layer of facia.

Innervation: Radial nerve (ALL!)

Superficial

The superficial layer muscles are all named *"extensor-"* except for the **brachioradialis**. Amongst the 5 *"extensor"* muscles, 3 are extensor *"carpi"* and 2 are extensor *"digit-"*.

From lateral to medial:

1. brachioradialis
2. extensor carpi radialis longus
3. extensor carpi radialis brevis
4. extensor digitorum
5. extensor digiti minimi
6. extensor carpi ulnaris

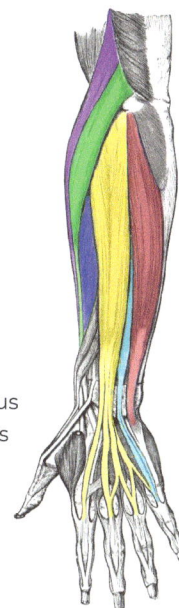

- ■ brachioradialis
- ■ extensor carpi radialis longus
- ■ extensor carpi radialis brevis
- ■ extensor digitorum
- ■ extensor digiti minimi
- ■ extensor carpi ulnaris

Deep

The deep layer has some funny-sounding names in it: a **snuffbox** (composed of 3 **policies** (*"pollicis"*)), an **indicis**, an **anaconda** (*anconeus*), and some **soup** (*supinator*). Think: *"if it sounds funny, it's probably in the deep layer."*

1. anconeus
2. supinator

Anatomical snuffbox
3. abductor pollicis longus ⎤
4. extensor pollicis brevis   ⎬ *"Brevis sandwich"*
5. extensor pollicis longus   ⎦
6. extensor indicis

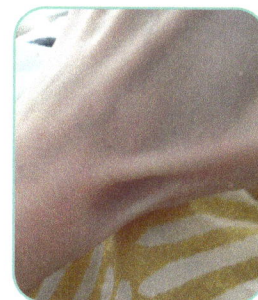

Do you even snuff, bro?

Remember: *"pollicis"* means *thumb*!

Anatomical snuffbox: The anatomical snuffbox is a triangular depression at the base of the thumb on the dorsum of the hand. The name originates from the use of this natural "box" to sniff *"snuff"* - a form of tobacco. It is clinically relevant because this area bears the brunt of the force when **falling on an outstretched hand**. It can fracture the **scaphoid** (most commonly fractured wrist bone), which causes **localized tenderness in the anatomical snuffbox**!

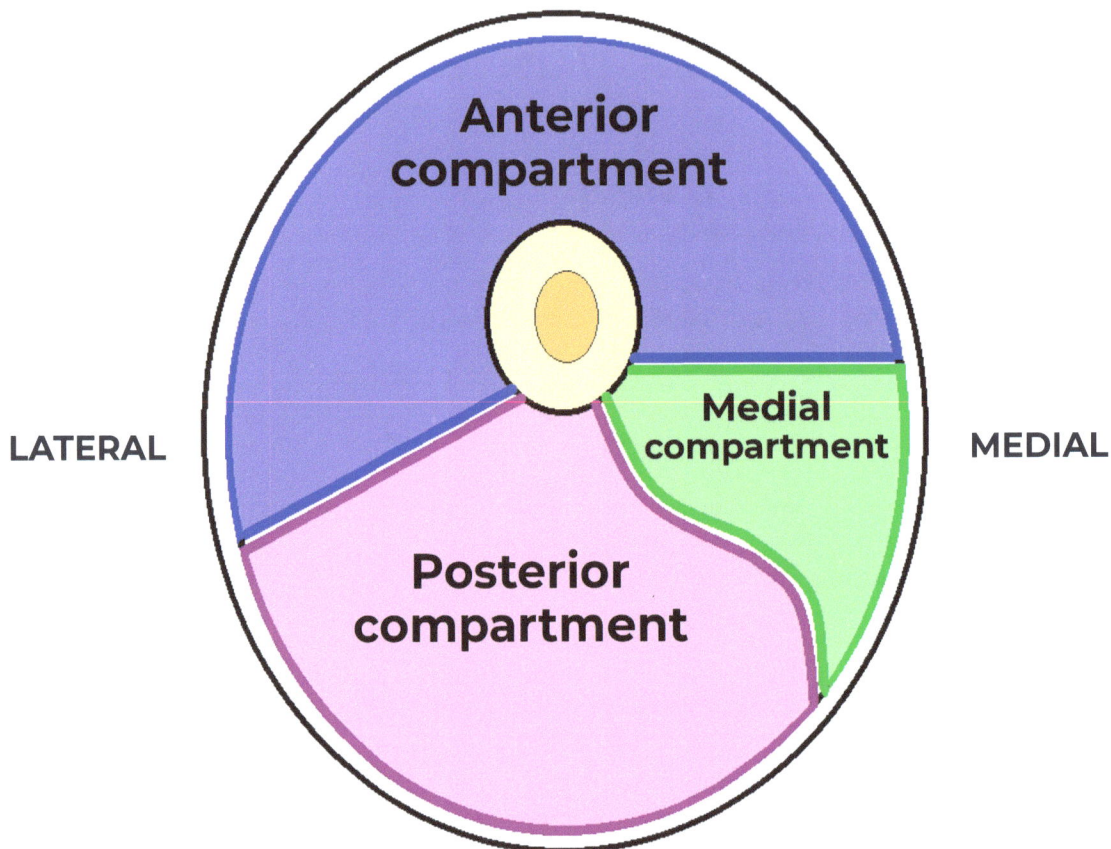

Anterior compartment

Medial compartment

LATERAL

MEDIAL

Posterior compartment

27 Thigh muscles

The muscles of each compartment all have the same general **function**, **blood supply**, and **innervation**.

A) Anterior compartment (3)
- **Quadriceps femoris, sartorius, pectineus**
  a. Innervation: **femoral nerve**
  b. Blood supply: **femoral artery**
  c. Function: **Flex thigh, extend knee**

B) Medial compartment (5)
- **3 adductors** (adductor magnus, longus, and brevis), **gracilis, obturator externus**
  a. Innervation: **obturator nerve**
  b. Blood supply: **obturator artery**
  c. Function: **Adduct thigh**

C) Posterior compartment (3)
- **Semitendinosus, semimembranosus, biceps femoris**
  a. Innervation: **sciatic nerve** (via its main branch, the tibial nerve)
  b. Blood supply: **profunda femoris artery, inferior gluteal artery**
  c. Function: **Extend thigh, flex knee**

❗ **Tip**: between semitendinosus & semimembranosus, semi**M**embranosus is the **M**edial one.

28 Lower leg muscles

The lower leg is separated by fascia into **4 compartments**: **anterior**, **lateral**, **superficial posterior**, and **deep posterior**. The muscles in each compartment have the same innervation.

MEDIAL

Tibia
Anterior
Lateral
Fibula
Deep Posterior
Superficial Posterior

Innervations:

- Anterior: **deep fibular (peroneal) nerve**
- Lateral: **superficial fibular (peroneal) nerve**
- Posterior (BOTH superficial and deep): **tibial nerve**

*All 3 nerves originate from the **sciatic nerve** (which splits into the tibial and common fibular nerves in the popliteal fossa just above the knee).

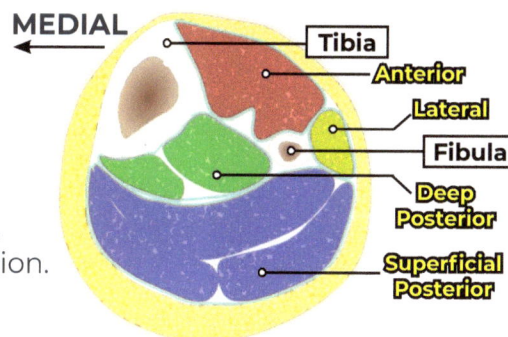

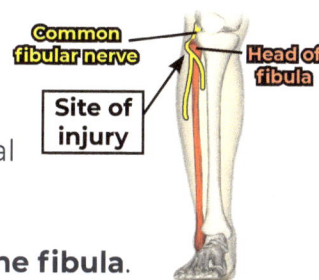

Common fibular nerve
Head of fibula
Site of injury

! The **common fibular nerve** commonly gets injured at the **head of the fibula**.

Lateral (2)

Start with the easiest first - the lateral compartment. At the lateral side of your leg is the **fibula**, so the two lateral compartment muscles must be named...

1. **Fibularis** longus
2. **Fibularis** brevis

Main function: eversion of foot

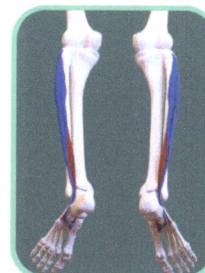

■ Fibularis longus
■ Fibularis brevis

Anterior (4) and Deep Posterior (4)

The anterior and deep posterior compartments are adjacent to each other and are **almost mirror images of each other**! They each have one muscle to act on the **foot**, one on the **digits (toes)**, one on the **big toe (hallux)**, and one **"P" muscle**.

	Anterior	Deep Posterior
Foot →	· tibialis anterior	· tibialis posterior
Toes →	· extensor digitorum longus	· flexor digitorum longus
Big toe →	· extensor hallucis longus	· flexor hallucis longus
"P" muscle →	· peroneus (fibularis) tertius	· popliteus

It makes sense that the extensors are anterior and flexors are posterior when you simply visualize the muscles as strings and imagine pulling on them. Alternatively, if in doubt, simply flex or extend your own foot and feel what muscles tighten up.

It makes sense that the **popliteus** is in the deep *posterior* compartment because the **popliteal fossa** is the space at the *posterior* of the knee.

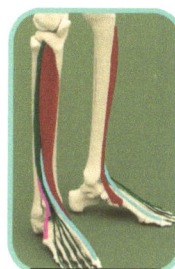

Anterior

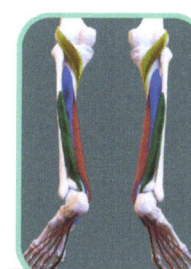

Deep Posterior

Superficial Posterior (3)

Think: **GPS** (see next page)

Superficial to deep: **1. Gastrocnemius, 2. Plantaris, 3. Soleus**

29 Superficial posterior lower leg muscles

GPS

The muscles of the superficial posterior lower leg are, from superficial to deep:

- **G**astrocnemius
- **P**lantaris
- **S**oleus

Visualize a **GPS** tracker that a convict wears around his **calf**.

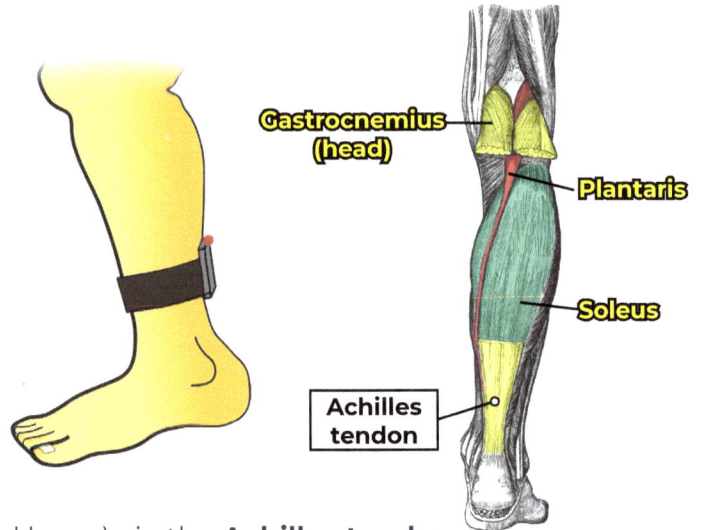

All 3 muscles insert onto the calcaneous (heel bone) via the **Achilles tendon**.

> ! The gastrocnemius and plantaris originate ABOVE the knee (i.e. in the femur), hence they can flex the knee. The soleus originates below the knee and cannot flex it.

Gastrocnemius (head)
Plantaris
Soleus
Achilles tendon

30 Lumbricals (of the hand)

The **L**umbricals make your hand an "**L**"

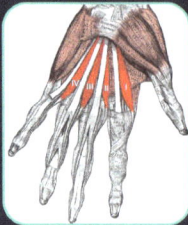

The lumbricals are one of 4 sets of intrinsic hand muscles (the other 3 being the **interossei**, **thenar**, and **hypothenar muscles**). They have 2 actions:

- **Flex metacarpophalangeal joints**
- **Extend interphalangeal joints**

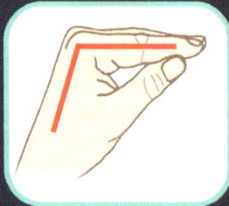

These two actions cause your hand to make an "**L**" shape.

31 Interosseous muscles of the hand

Palmar = ADduct
Dorsal = ABduct

PAD/DAB

Palmar: **AD**ducts
Dorsal: **AB**ducts

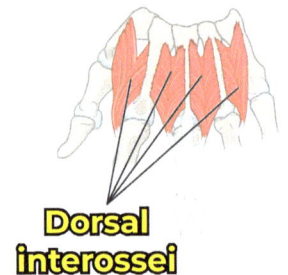

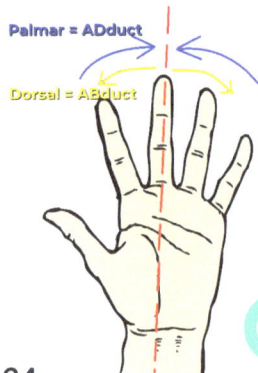

Dorsal interossei

The name *Inter-osseous* tells you they are *between* the *bones* of your hand (i.e. 5 metacarpals), and therefore must move them from side to side.

> ! Both interossei are innervated by the **ulnar nerve** (remember: the intrinsic hand muscles are ALL innervated by the ulnar nerve except the 'LOAF' muscles).

32 Intrinsic foot muscles

2 dorsal, 10 plantar (in 4 layers)

Intrinsic foot muscles are divided into **dorsal** and **plantar** muscles. The dorsal side is extremely simple, having just 2 muscles. The 10 plantar muscles however are divided into 4 layers.

Innervations
Dorsal muscles: **Deep fibular nerve**
Plantar muscles: **Tibial nerve** (via medial and lateral *plantar* nerves)

Dorsal

Just 2 extensors:

1. **extensor** digitorum brevis
2. **extensor** hallucis brevis

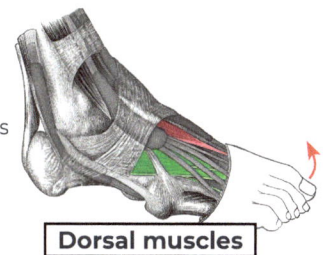

🟩 Extensor digitorum brevis
🟥 Extensor hallucis brevis

Dorsal muscles

- These two muscles are simply the *"brevis"* versions of the *extensor digitorum longus* and *extensor hallucis longus* that are found just superiorly in the anterior compartment of the lower leg.

- As with the lower leg extensors, it makes sense that the foot extensors are on the dorsal surface (i.e. *top* of the foot) so that they can pull the toes *up* (= extension).

Plantar

Layers 1 to 4 are numbered from superficial to deep:

Layers 1 and 3: *almost* **mirror images of each other.**

Layer 1	Layer 3
· abductor hallucis	· adductor hallucis
· flexor digitorum brevis	· flexor hallucis brevis
· abductor digiti minimi	· flexor digiti minimi brevis

Layer 2: 2 muscles

1. **lumbricals**
2. quadratus **plantae**

Picture **2 lumber**jacks chopping down a **plant**.

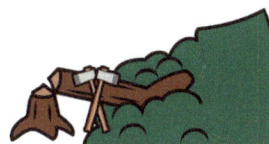

Layer 4: just **2 interossei muscles** (**dorsal** and **plantar**)

- There are 4 dorsal and 3 plantar interossei (just like in the hand!)
- It makes sense that the interossei muscles are in the deepest layer, as the name **inter-ossei** tells you they're **in between** the **bones** (metatarsals).

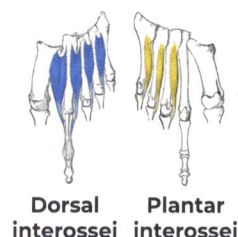

Dorsal   Plantar
interossei interossei

33 Muscles of mastication (chewing)

There are 4 muscles of mastication:

1. **Lateral pterygoid**
2. **Medial pterygoid**
3. **Temporalis**
4. **Masseter**

> **L**ateral pterygoid
> **L**owers the jaw

The lateral pterygoid is the only one beginning with "**L**", and likewise is the only one that **L**owers the jaw – the other 3 elevating it.

Tip: When you clench your jaw, you can feel your **temporalis** flexing at your **temple** and your **masseter** (or *"mass-eater"*) flexing at the **angle of your jaw**. The two pterygoids are deeper and harder to feel.

Innervation: As all 4 muscles function to move the **mandible** up or down, all 4 are innervated by the **mandibular nerve** (a branch of **CN 5**). This is in contrast to most *facial* muscles, which are innervated by the *facial* nerve.

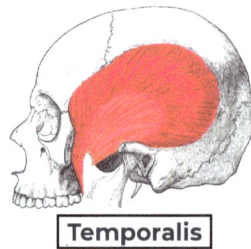

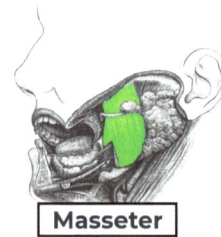

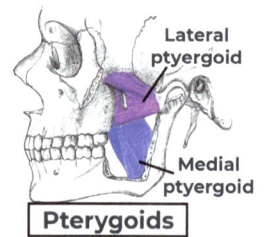

Temporalis | **Masseter** | **Pterygoids**

Lateral ptyergoid
Medial ptyergoid

34 Muscle fiber types

> **1 SLOW RED OX**

1 = type 1 fiber
slow = slow twitch
red = red fibers due to high mitochondria & myoglobin concentrations
ox = high oxidative phosphorylation

Then simply remember Type 2 fibers are the opposite (*fast, white, & more anaerobic*)

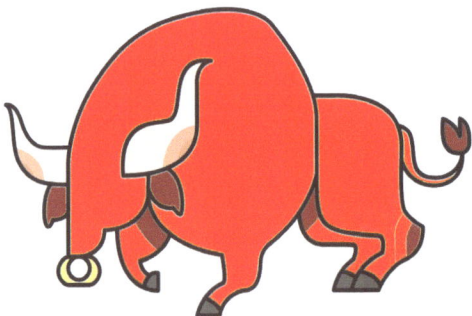

Alternative: Simply remember the **speed** of Type 1 and Type 2 fibers, and the rest can be logically deduced. Slow fibers (think marathon runners) must last long, so they use oxidative phosphorylation (an aerobic process). Hence they require myoglobin & mitochondria. Hence they're RED!

Dr.You
METHOD

35 Rotator cuff muscles

ANTERIOR side

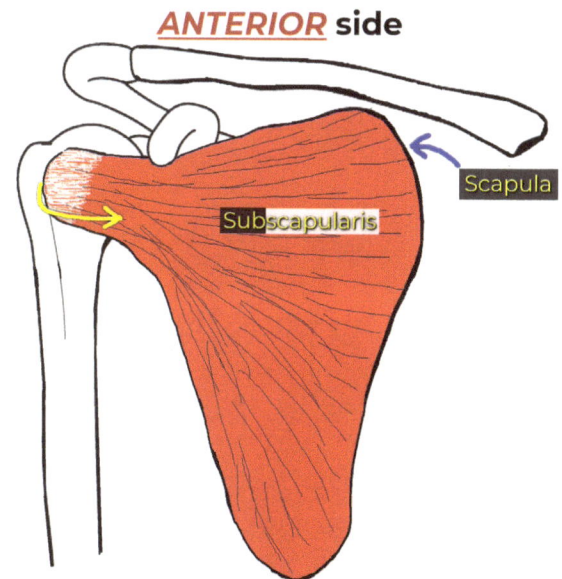

Scapula

Subscapularis

SITS

Supraspinatus
Infraspinatus
Teres minor
Subscapularis

IN THE NAME!

Locations: There's only one rotator cuff muscle that sits on the anterior side of the scapula. *Hint* - it's *in the name*: it's the **sub-scapularis**. The rest lie on the posterior side. The **supra-spinatus** lies **above** the **spine** of the scapula and the **infra-spinatous** below it, as their names imply.

Posterior side

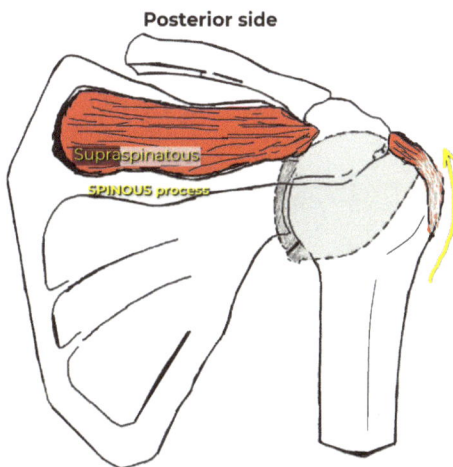

Supraspinatous

SPINOUS process

Posterior side

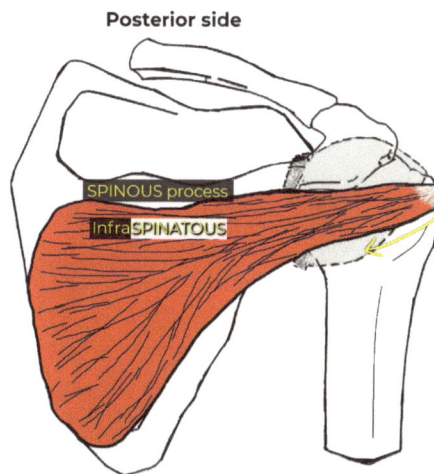

SPINOUS process

InfraSPINATOUS

Posterior side

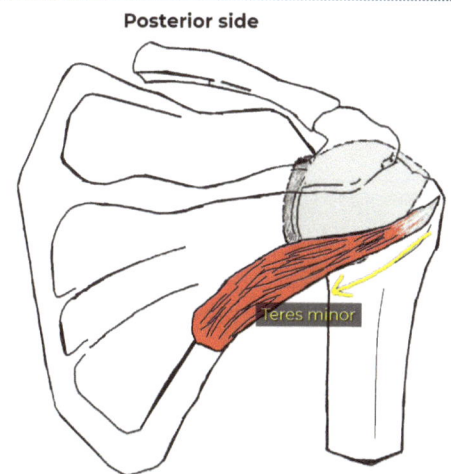

Teres minor

FUNCTIONS

All 4 rotator cuff muscles insert onto the lateral part of the humerus. With that in mind, their functions can all easily be deduced by remembering that the subscapularis is the only one lying anteriorly and the rest lying posteriorly – then simply imagining what happens if you pull on the muscle:

- **Subscapularis**: only one that internally rotates the arm
- **Infraspinatus** and **teres minor**: externally rotate the arm
- **Supraspinatus**: name tells you it lies superiorly - hence lifts up (abducts) the arm

TESTS
- **Supraspinatus**: Empty Can test, Drop Arm test
- **Infraspinatus** and **teres minor**: simple external rotation
- **Subscapularis**: Lift Off test, Bear-Hug test

36 Muscles of elbow flexion

The 3 B's Bend the elbow

Biceps brachii
Brachialis
Brachioradialis

Alternatively, you can think of the **3 'brachi'.**

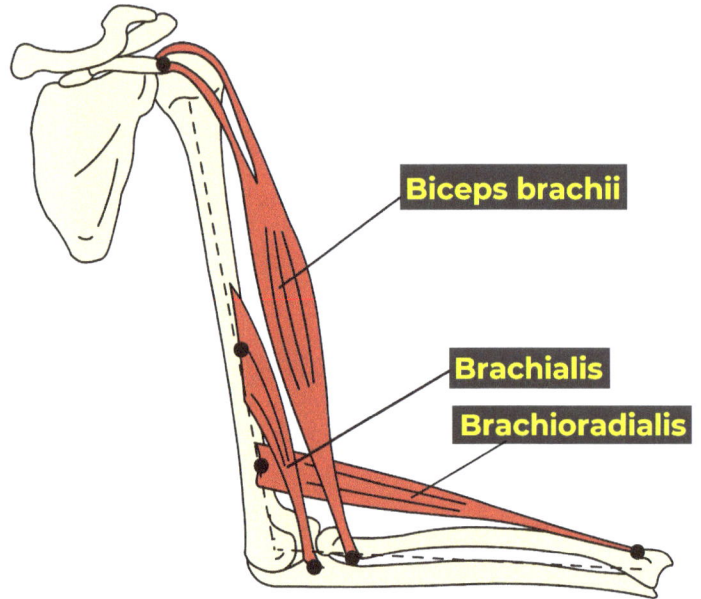

Biceps brachii

Brachialis
Brachioradialis

IN THE NAME! To remember the location of each muscle, think of its name. The majority of the brachio**radialis** spans the **radius**. The majority of the **brachialis** (*brachi/brachium* meaning **upper arm**) spans the **brachium**. Everyone knows where the biceps brachii is.

37 Extrinsic tongue muscles

1st part of name: muscle origin
2nd part of name (-*glossus* for ALL): attaches onto tongue

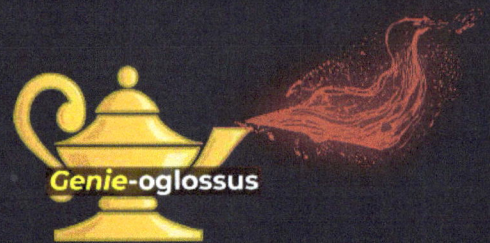

Genie-oglossus

Knowing the origin and attachment, each muscle's function can then be deduced by simply imagining what would happen if you pulled on it.

1. **Hyoglossus:** brings tongue back to **hyoid** bone (**retraction**)
2. **Styloglossus** & 3. **palatoglossus**: lift tongue up towards **palate** and **styloid process** (**elevation**)
4. **Genioglossus:** protrudes tongue out towards **chin** ('**genio-**'), like a **genie coming out of a bottle**

38 External vs. internal abdominal obliques

Make an "X" with your arms over your belly - this is the direction of the eXternal oblique muscle

(internal obliques run opposite to that)

Near the midline of your abdomen, you have only one major muscle: the **rectus abdominis** (your "6-pack" muscles). However as you move laterally, you have 3 layers of muscles (from superficial to deep):

*   **External oblique**
*   **Internal oblique** (perpendicular to external oblique)
*   **Transversus abdominis** (completely horizontal)

As these 3 muscles approach the rectus abdominis, they become aponeuroses (broad, flat tendons), which then wrap around the rectus abdominis like a sheath. This sheath is cleverly named the **rectus sheath** (see *Layers of the Abdominal Wall* mnemonic in the GI chapter).

All 4 of these abdominal muscles are accessory muscles of **EXPIRATION** - they help perform **forced exhalation**. This is because they all squeeze the abdomen, which increases its pressure. This causes the abdominal organs to push upward against the diaphragm and lungs, squeezing air out.

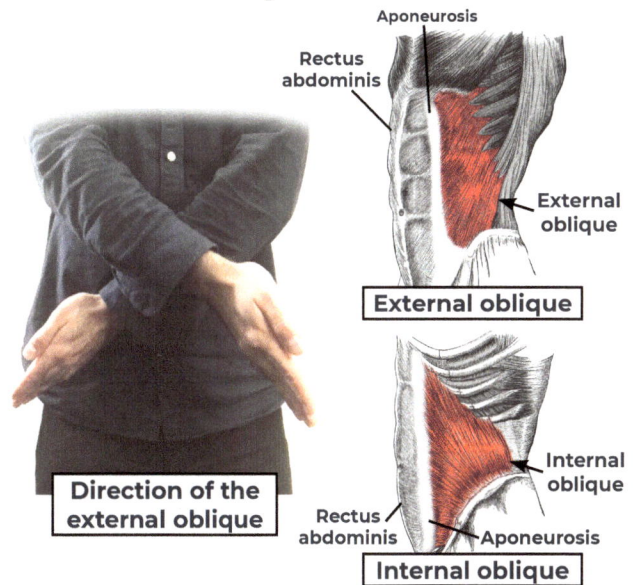

Direction of the external oblique

Aponeurosis
Rectus abdominis
External oblique
External oblique

Internal oblique
Rectus abdominis
Aponeurosis
Internal oblique

39 Anterior vs. posterior cruciate ligaments

Make the same "X" with your arms as the previous mnemonic except over your right knee

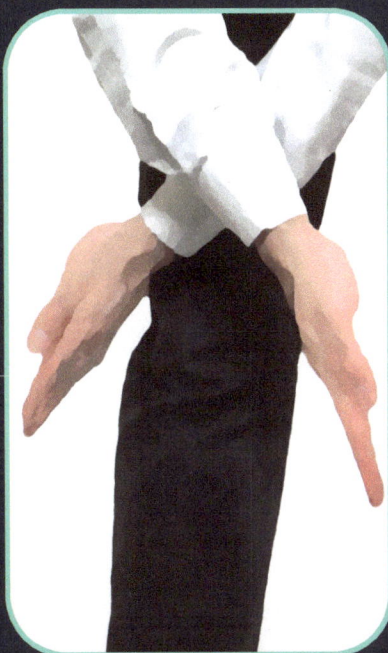

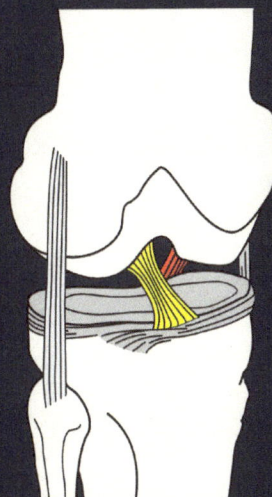

With your right arm anterior to your left, your **anterior** arm runs in the same direction as your **anterior** cruciate ligament (ACL) and your **posterior** arm in the same direction as your **posterior** cruciate ligament (PCL).

Tests for ligament injury

*   **Anterior** cruciate ligament: **Anterior drawer test**

*   **Posterior** cruciate ligament: **Posterior drawer test**

Right knee, anterior view
■ ACL
■ PCL

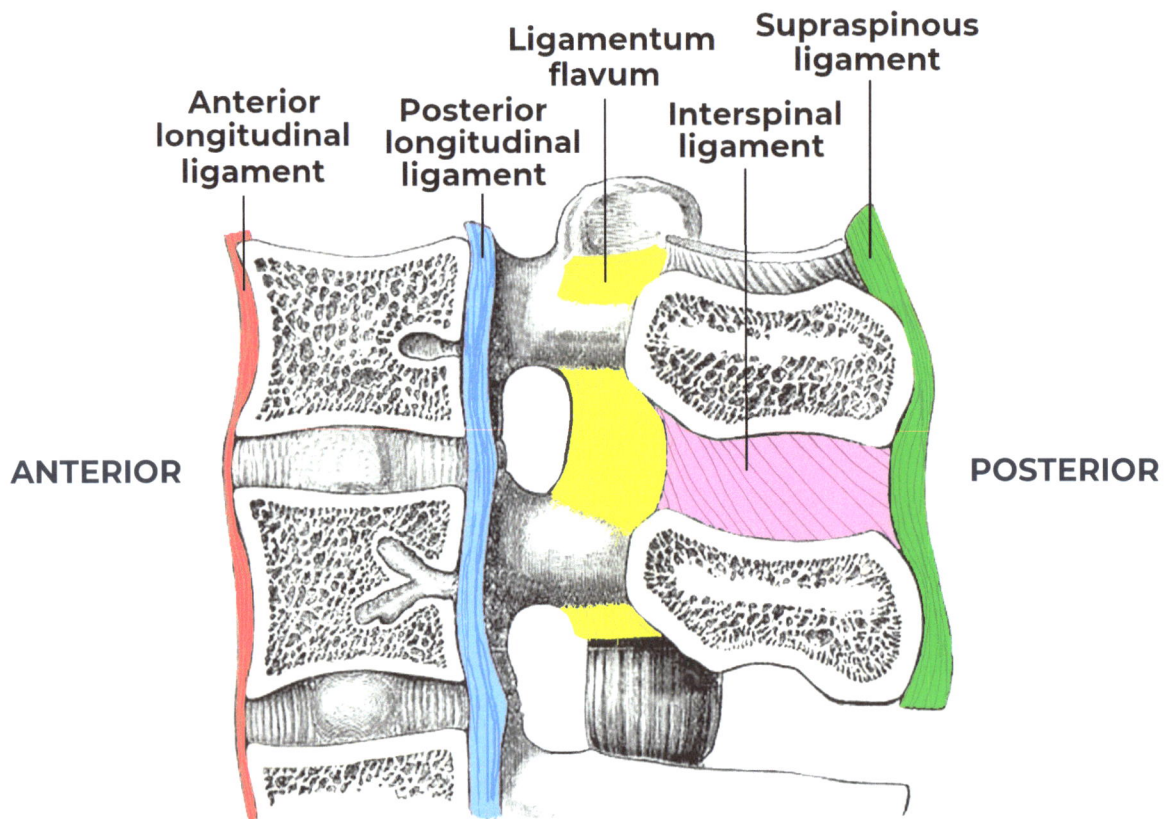

Anterior longitudinal ligament

Posterior longitudinal ligament

Ligamentum flavum

Interspinal ligament

Supraspinous ligament

ANTERIOR

POSTERIOR

40 Spinal ligaments

It's in the name

IN THE NAME!

There are **5** major spinal ligaments. They are, from superficial to deep:

1. Supraspinous ligaments
- The name '**supra-spinous**' literally tells you it is "**above**" (i.e. **outside**) the **spine**

2. Interspinal ligament
- Again, the name '**inter-spinal**' tells you it lies **between** the **spine** (i.e. between spinous processes of vertebrae)

3. Ligamentum flava
- The ligamentum **flava** can taste the **flava** of the epidural space, as it is the layer immediately outside of the epidural space and dura mater of the spinal cord

4. Posterior longitudinal ligament
- The **posterior** longitudinal ligament lies immediately **posterior** to the spine

5. Anterior longitudinal ligament
- The **anterior** longitudinal ligament lies immediately **anterior** to the spine

(!) Since the **ligamentum flava** is right outside the epidural space, it's used as a landmark when performing **epidural anesthesia**. When you penetrate it, you feel a "pop" (loss of resistance), which tells you you're in the epidural space.

CHAPTER 5

Peripheral Nerves

41 Master list of nerve roots

The following is a table containing important nerves in the body and their roots:

Nerve	Roots
Phrenic	C3 - C5
Axillary	C5 - C6
Musculocutaneous	C5 - C7
Long thoracic nerve	C5 - C7
Radial	C5 - T1
Median	C5 - T1
Ulnar	C8 - T1
Iliohypogastric	T12 - L1
Genitofemoral	L1 - L2
Lateral cutaneous nerve	L2 - L3
Obturator	L2 - L4
Femoral	L2 - L4
Saphenous (branch of femoral)	L3 - L4
Sciatic	L4 - S3
Common peroneal (fibular)	L4 - S2
Tibial	L4 - S3
Superior Gluteal	L4 - S1
Inferior gluteal	L5 - S2
Pudendal	S2 - S4

Upper extremity (Axillary through Ulnar)

Lower extremity (Iliohypogastric through Pudendal)

Fill in more as you go

42 Trendelenburg sign

A _trendy_ new way to walk for those who think they're _superior_.

Trendelenburg sign is when there's a lesion of the **superior gluteal nerve**, causing the contralateral side of the hip to sag.

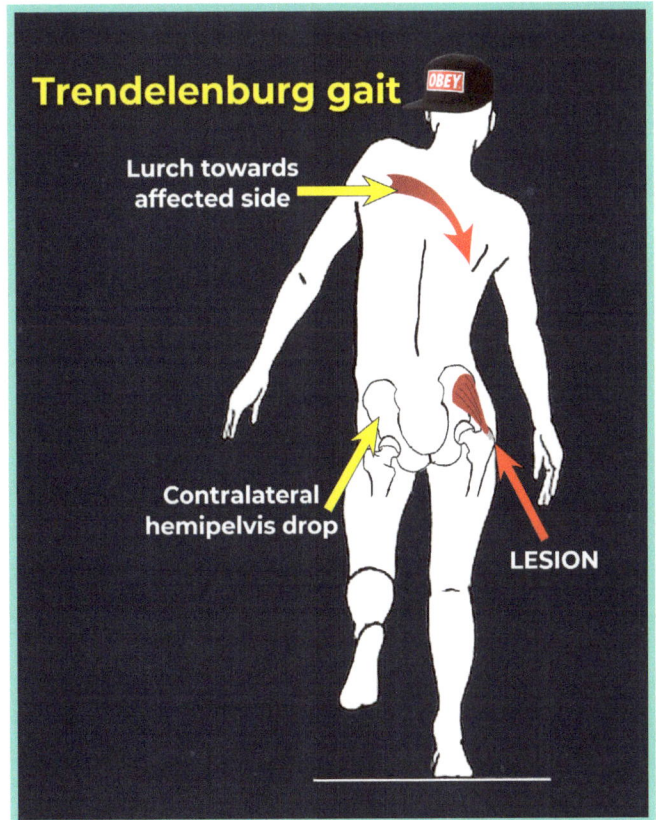

Trendelenburg gait

Lurch towards affected side

Contralateral hemipelvis drop

LESION

OBEY

! Remember that it's the side of the hip **OPPOSITE** to the lesion that sags because walking with such arrogance is truly **OPPOSITE** to the way a good person walks.

43 Superior vs. inferior gluteal nerve

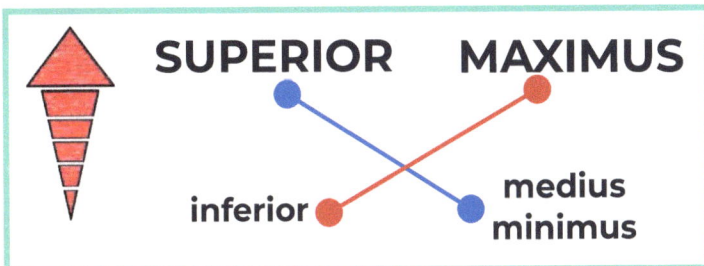

SUPERIOR   MAXIMUS

inferior   medius minimus

Simply think of the "magnitudes" of the names and remember that they innervate the OPPOSITE of their magnitude:

- **SUPERIOR** gluteal nerve innervates the gluteus **MINIMUS** & **MEDIUS**
- **INFERIOR** gluteal nerve innervates the gluteus **MAXIMUS**

44 Sensory innervation of the ear

> **All in the name (+ V for Vagus)**
>
> IN THE NAME!

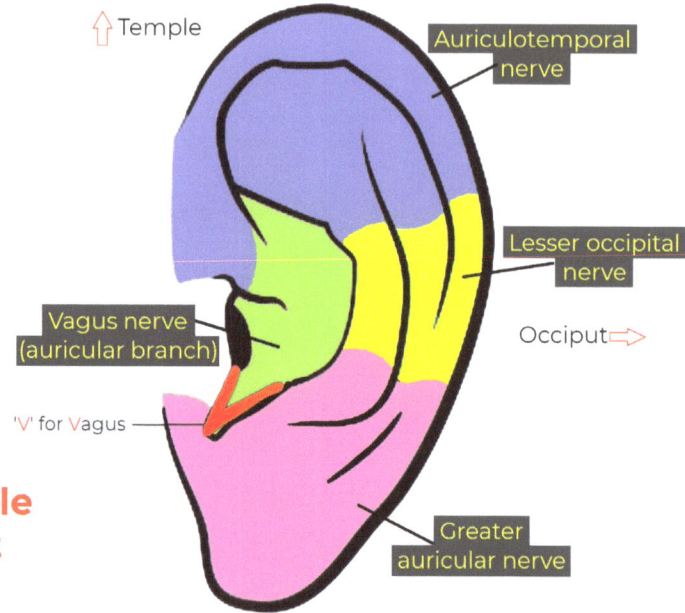

Temple

Auriculotemporal nerve

Lesser occipital nerve

Occiput ⇨

Vagus nerve (auricular branch)

'V' for Vagus

Greater auricular nerve

4 parts:
1. **Auriculotemporal**: by the **temple**
2. **Lesser occipital**: by the **occiput**
3. **Vagus**: find the '**V**'
4. **Greater auricular**: the remaining area

45 Tendon reflexes

> **Sign the rhyme**

<u>**Achilles reflex: S1, S2**</u> *("buckle my shoe")*
<u>**Patellar reflex: L3, L4**</u> *("kick the door")*
<u>**Biceps and brachioradialis reflexes: C5, C6**</u> *("pick up sticks")*
<u>**Triceps reflex: C7, C8**</u> *("lay them straight")*

(!) **Remember:** deep tendon reflexes don't go to the brain. They're simply loops between the tendon, spinal cord, and muscle. That's why they can even be present after brain death has occured!

> **Grading**
> 0 - absent
> +1 - diminished
> **+2 - normal**
> +3 - hyperactive
> +4 - hyperactive with clonus

<u>**Motor neuron lesions:**</u> From the brain to the muscle, there are two motor neurons - the first one (e.g. from the brain to the spinal cord) is called an **upper motor neuron (UMN)**, and the second (e.g. spinal cord to the muscle) is called a **lower motor neuron (LMN)**. A lesion to an UMN causes **hyperreflexia**, while a lesion to a LMN causes **hyporeflexia**. This makes sense because a LMN can still fire in the absence of an UMN (via other stimuli), but if a LMN is not intact, there is nothing to make the muscle contract.

Dr.You
METHOD

46 Drawing the brachial plexus

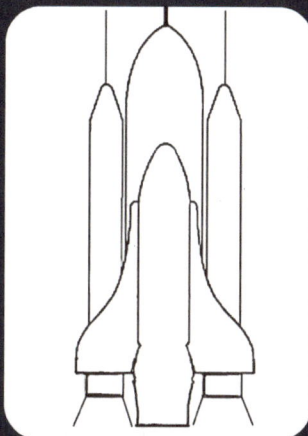

Draw a **rocket ship**

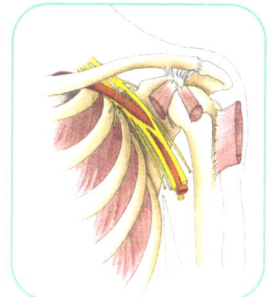

What even is the brachial plexus?
The brachial plexus is a web-like network of nerves that starts in the neck and travels through the armpit and down the arm. It gives rise to the 5 major nerves of the upper extremity (**axillary, musculocutaneous, radial, median,** and **ulnar**), which supply the upper extremity with both sensory (afferent) and and motor (efferent) innervation. The plexus is formed by the roots of the **C5, C6, C7, C8,** and **T1** nerves.

Brachial plexus
(everything in yellow)

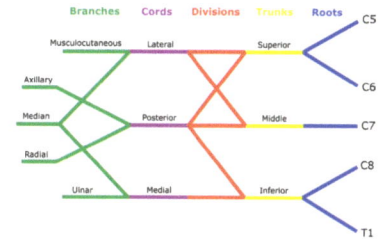

The details of the plexus's interconnections are sometimes tested on. Therefore, practice drawing it out. To do so, draw a rocket ship in 4 steps:

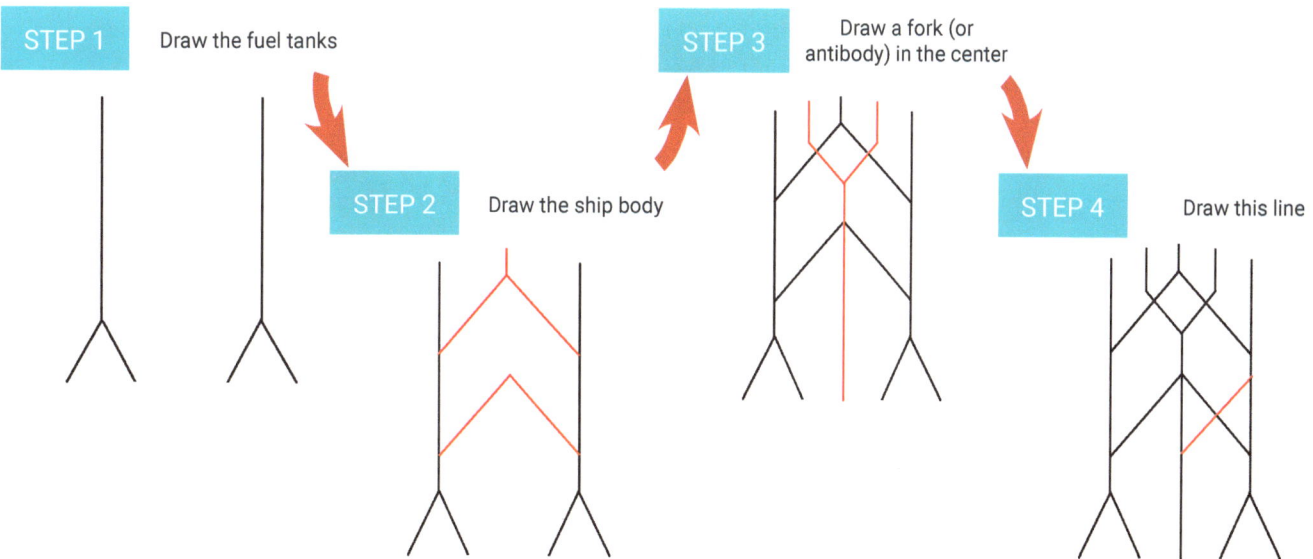

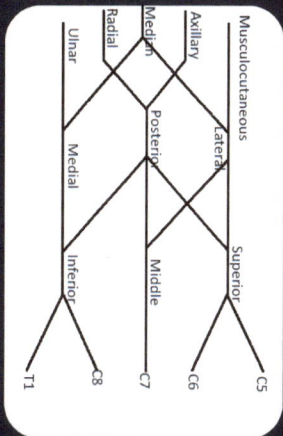

STEP 1 Draw the fuel tanks

STEP 2 Draw the ship body

STEP 3 Draw a fork (or antibody) in the center

STEP 4 Draw this line

Brachial plexus

Rocket ship

BONUS: Draw a **long** fuel leak from the right fuel tank (the **long thoracic nerve** from **C5, C6,** & **C7**):

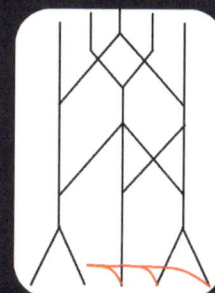

47 Brachial plexus sections

Follow the divisions of a **tree** - the brachial plexus is named similarly!

The sections are:

1. Roots
2. Trunk
3. Divisions
4. Cords
5. Branches

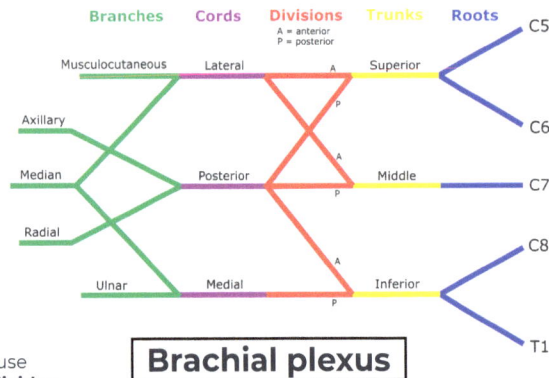

Tip: **Divisions** are named so because that is where the plexus literally **divides**...

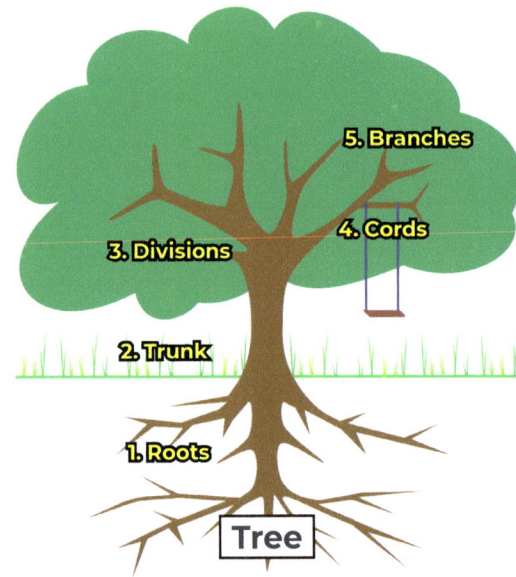

Brachial plexus

Branches	Cords	Divisions	Trunks	Roots
Musculocutaneous	Lateral	A = anterior, P = posterior	Superior	C5, C6
Axillary				
Median	Posterior		Middle	C7
Radial				
Ulnar	Medial		Inferior	C8, T1

Tree

5. Branches
4. Cords
3. Divisions
2. Trunk
1. Roots

48 Diaphragm innervation

"C3-5 keeps the diaphragm **alive!"**

The diaphragm is the **principle muscle of respiration** and is innervated by the **phrenic nerve** (which originates from C3-5).

49 Median nerve innervation of intrinsic hand muscles

A **medium**-sized **LOAF** of bread

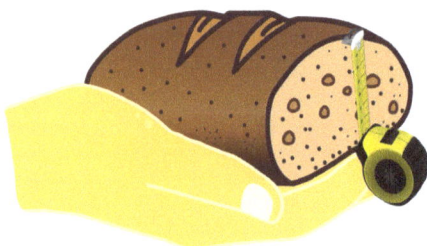

The **ulnar nerve** innervates all intrinsic hand muscles except:

Lumbricals (lateral two)
Opponens pollicis
Abductor pollicis brevis
Flexor pollicis brevis

These are innervated by the **median** ("*medium*") nerve

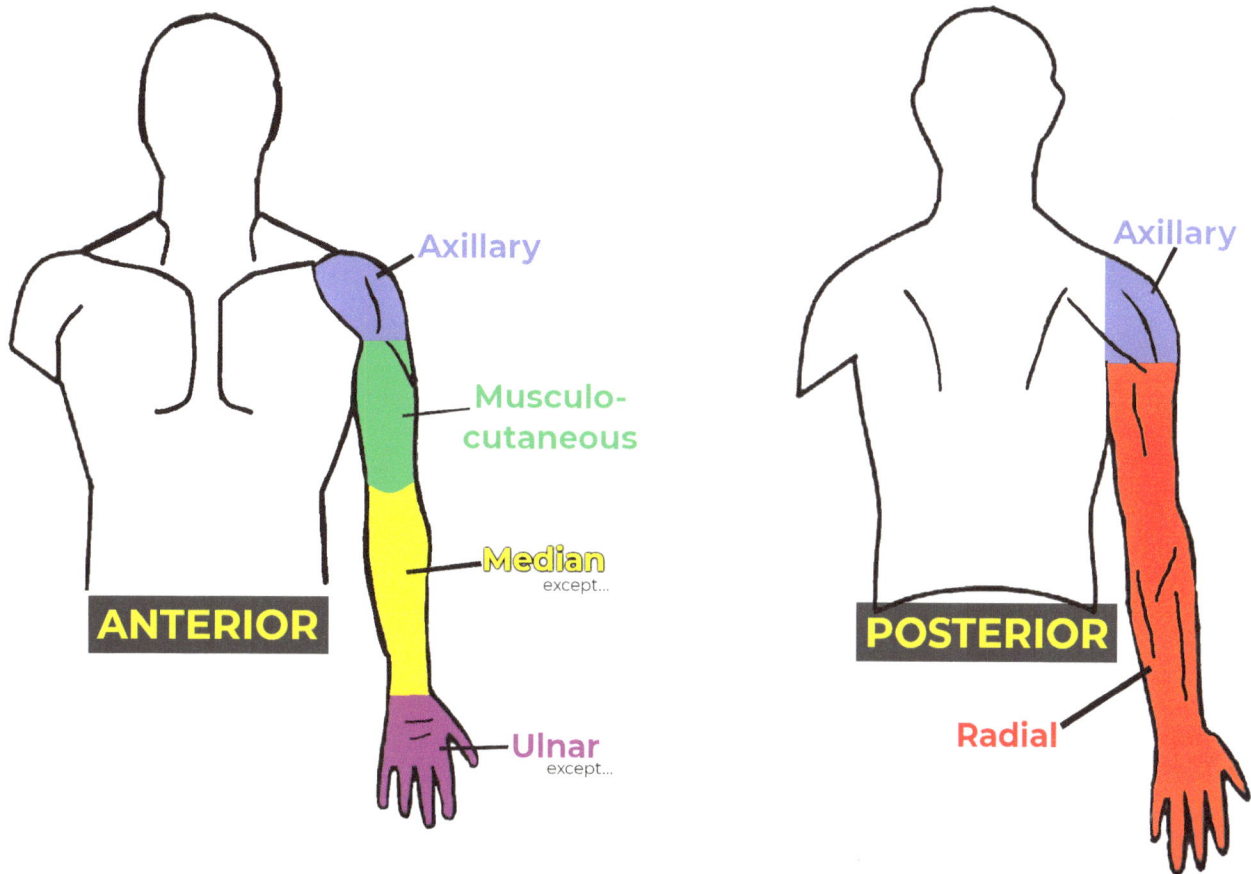

Dr.You
METHOD

Axillary

Musculo-cutaneous

Median
except...

ANTERIOR

Ulnar
except...

Axillary

POSTERIOR

Radial

50 Motor innervation of upper extremities

The motor innervation of the upper extremities, if mentally well-organized, can be very easy to remember:

Shoulder (deltoids): **axillary** nerve (appropriately named, as it's by the **axilla**)

Anterior side:
- **Upper arm:** **musculo**cutaneous nerve (**muscle**-men like to flex their biceps)
- **Forearm:** **median nerve** for all except two that are innervated by the ulnar nerve:
  - 1. flexor carpi ulnaris
  - 2. flexor digitorum profundus [medial two parts] ("profoundly different innervation")
- **Hand:** **ulnar nerve** for all except the 4 *'LOAF'* muscles, which are innervated by the median nerve (see *LOAF* mnemonic)

Posterior side:
- Excluding the shoulder, the **radial nerve** innervates **ALL** of the extensor muscles of the upper extremity

COMMON NERVE INJURY LOCATIONS

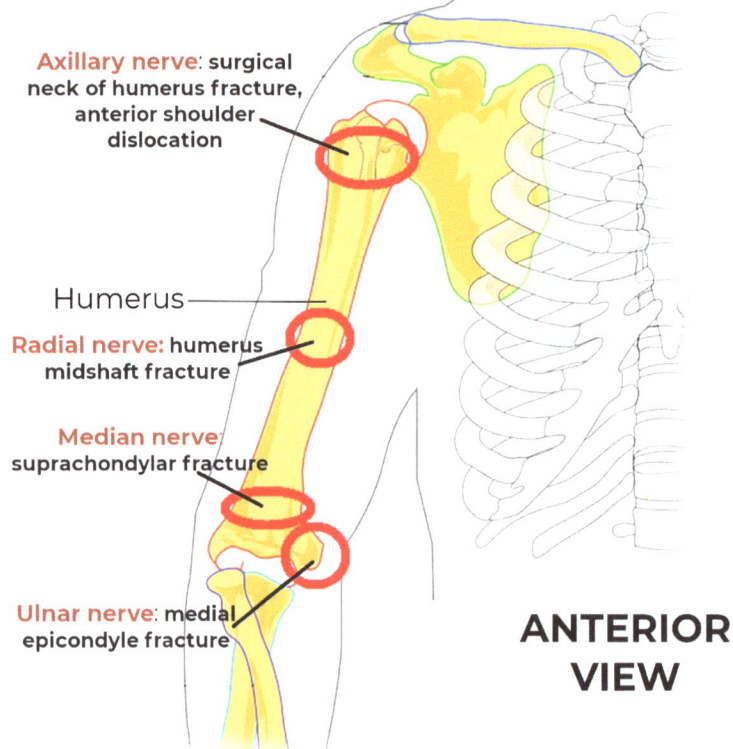

Axillary nerve: surgical neck of humerus fracture, anterior shoulder dislocation

Humerus

Radial nerve: humerus midshaft fracture

Median nerve: suprachondylar fracture

Ulnar nerve: medial epicondyle fracture

ANTERIOR VIEW

51 Common injury locations of arm nerves

1. Axillary nerve: surgical neck of humerus fracture and anterior shoulder dislocation
- makes sense as the **axillary** nerve remains in the **axilla** and doesn't travel far down the arm

2. Radial nerve: humerus midshaft fracture
- the **radial nerve** travels along the back of the humerus ("**radiates** away from you"), hence it can be injured by a break in the humerus midshaft

3. Median nerve: suprachondylar fracture
- the **median nerve** gets injured right around the **middle** of the arm

4. Ulnar nerve: medial epicondyle fracture
- makes sense as the ulnar nerve travels along the medial side of the arm ("**ulnar nerve** gets injured right above the **ulna**")

CHAPTER 6

Bones

52 Long bone terminology

Physis: where new bone fuses

Long bones can be divided into 4 segments, all of whose names revolve around the **growth plate** (the *"physis"*):

1. **Physis:** growth plate (only found in children/adolescents)
2. **Epi**physis: "part **above** the physis" - the rounded end part that makes up the joint
3. **Diaphysis:** main shaft
4. **Meta**physis: "**middle**-physis" - in the **middle** of the epiphysis and diaphysis

Diaphysis

Physis would be around here in a growing person | Metaphysis

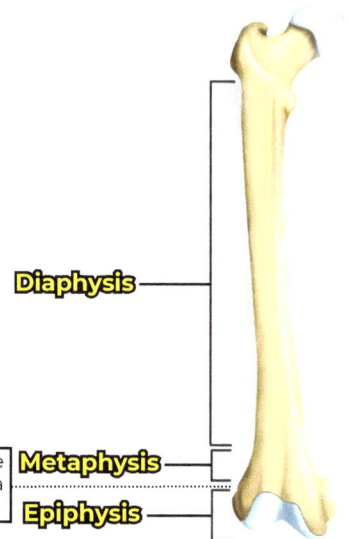

Epiphysis

Remember: not only is the **physis** where new bone "fuses", but the very physis itself literally **fuses** when adulthood is reached (called **growth plate fusion**) and is then called the *epiphysial line*.

On X-ray, the long bones of a growing person can look "**fractured**" at their ends. These are just the growth plates, and since they're made of cartilage they don't show up as bright on X-ray. They're not actual fractures!

Real fractures *can* involve the growth plate though, and they're called **Salter-Harris fractures**. They can actually disrupt normal growth and cause a person to be shorter on one side.

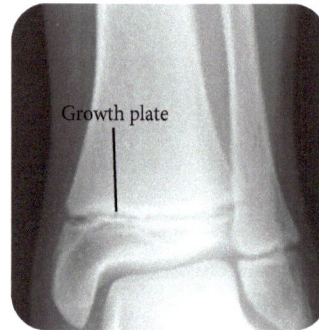

Growth plate

Normal child's tibia/ fibula X-ray

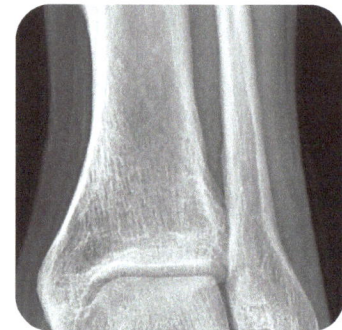

Normal adult's tibia/ fibula X-ray

53 Carpal vs. tarsal bones

- **Carpal: think "carpenter" or remember carpal tunnel syndrome**
- **Tarsal: the other one**

Carpal and tarsal - two similar words, both similar in function. They're easy to confuse, so remember:

- **Carpal**: located in the **hand**
- **Tarsal**: located in the **foot**

Carpenters work with their *carpal* bones (i.e. hands). You can also think "Tarsal - Toes" (while remembering they're not actually the toe bones!)

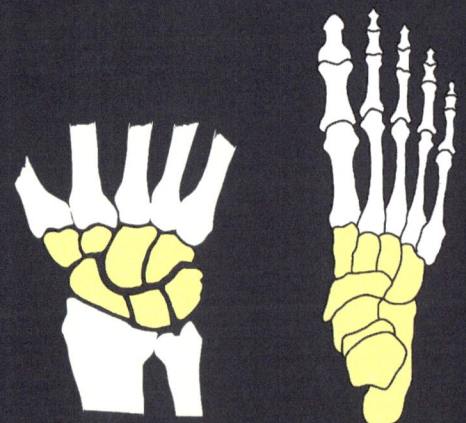

Carpal bones

Tarsal bones

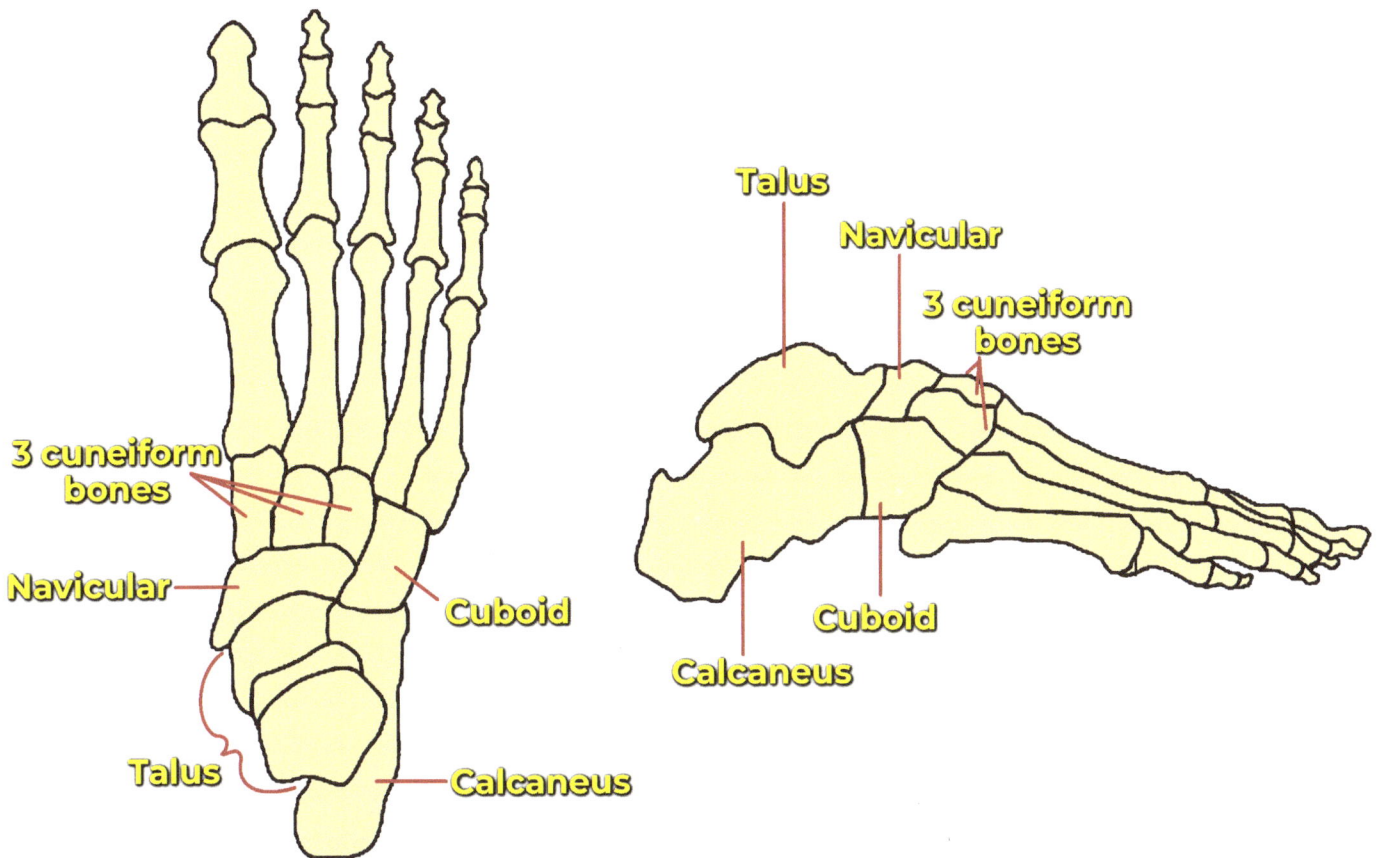

Talus

Navicular

3 cuneiform bones

3 cuneiform bones

Navicular

Cuboid

Cuboid

Calcaneus

Talus

Calcaneus

54 **Tarsal bones of the foot**

1. **Calcaneus:** heel
2. **Talus:** the "*tallest*" bone (i.e. most superior)
3. **3 Cuneiform bones:** lined up in *uniform* (i.e. tells you there's a few of them and they're lined up together)
4. **Navicular:** stuck in a **peculiar** position in the middle of 3 arguing cuneiform bones
5. **Cuboid:** literally is shaped like a **cube**; way off to the side in its own little cuboid universe

(!) The most commonly fractured tarsal bones are the **calcaneus** and **talus** - usually due to a fall from a height. This makes sense becaues the tibia - and hence all of your weight - lies directly over these two bones.

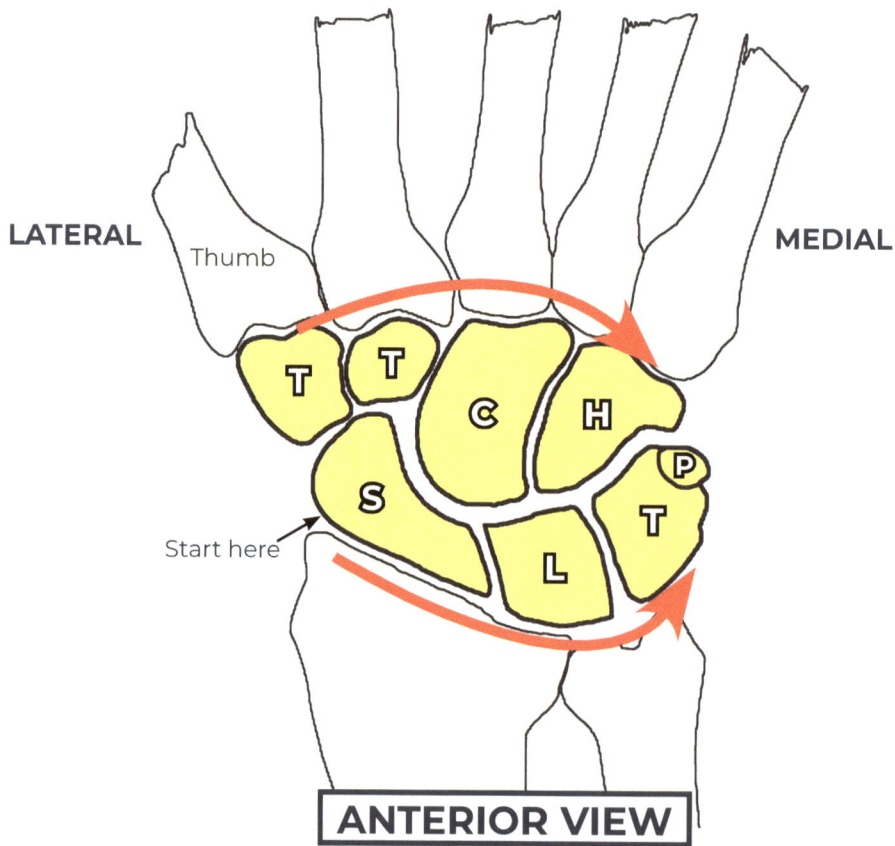

LATERAL   Thumb   MEDIAL

Start here

ANTERIOR VIEW

55 **Carpal (wrist) bones**

Sweet **L**ittle **T**ip: **P**ractice **T**hose **T**hings **C**alled **H**andbones

Here's a sweet little tip for learning anatomy: __practice__ makes perfect! Coincidentally, that also gives rise to a great mnemonic for __those things called "handbones"__ (i.e. carpal bones), moving medially from the scaphoid:

Scaphoid
Lunate
Triquetrum
Pisiform
Trapezium
Trapezoid
Capitate
Hamate

(!) Most commonly injured: **scaphoid** (falling on outstretched hand)
- Stretch out your hand and imagine falling - it makes sense!
- Can result in **avascular necrosis** (bone dies from lack of blood) due to its retrograde blood flow (= easier to block the blood supply)

(!) **Lunate dislocations** may injure the **median nerve**, causing **carpal tunnel syndrome**
- Makes sense, as it's right in the middle, which is where the median nerve travels (hence the name 'median')

(!) The trapezium and the trapezoid are easy to confuse, so remember that they appear in alphabetical order (**trapezium** before **trapezoid**).

56 — Osteoblasts vs. osteoclasts

> **OsteoBlasts: Build bone (with Base).**
> **OsteoClasts: Crush bone (with acid)**

Osteoblasts are the cells that build new bone. They do so under basic conditions.
Osteoclasts are the cells that break down bone (resorption). They do so by secreting acid.

57 — Bones of the arm and forearm

Arm
- **Humerus**: contains at its bottom the "**funny bone**" (or shall we say, the '*humorous*' bone?)

Forearm
- **Radius**: *radiates* away from you (i.e. lateral of the two when in anatomical position)
- Ulna: the other one

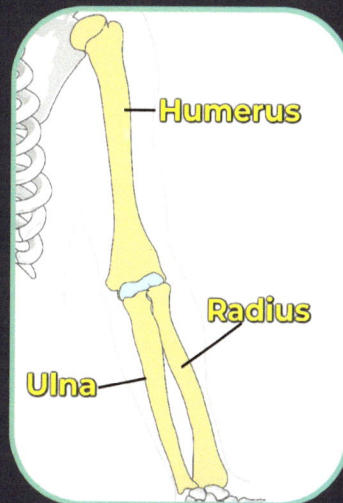

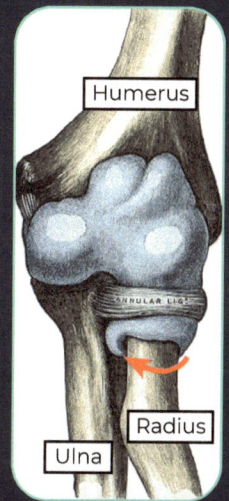

(!) **Radius rotates:** Your **radius** is the one that **rotates** and turns over, while your ulna is fixed to the humerus. This means that any muscle that rotates the forearm MUST attach to the radius! This is because the humeroulnar joint is a simple **hinge joint**, allowing only flexion/extension, while the humeroradial joint is a **ball-and-socket joint**, which rotates.

58 — Acromion vs. coracoid processes

> **Acromion = Above; Attaches to clavicle**

BOTH the acromion and coracoid processes are **part of the scapula** and serve to **stabilize the shoulder joint**. The acromion process lies superiorly and articulates with the **clavicle** to form the **acromioclavicular joint**. The coracoid process is a little worm-like hook that serves as the **attachment site for 3 muscles** (**coraco**brachialis, pectoralis minor, biceps brachii [short head]). Just look at it - doesn't it look like a great hook for muscles?

Alternative: think "acromi-**on-top**" ('*acro*-' literally means *highest*)

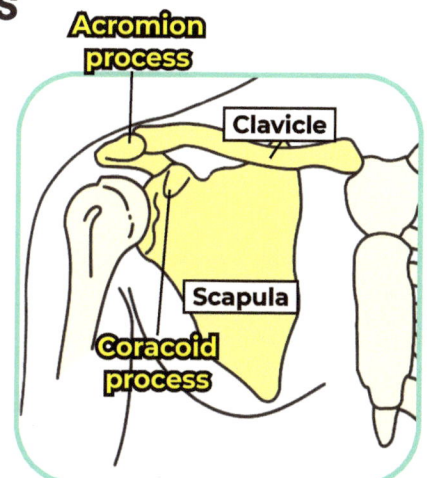

Anterior view of shoulder.

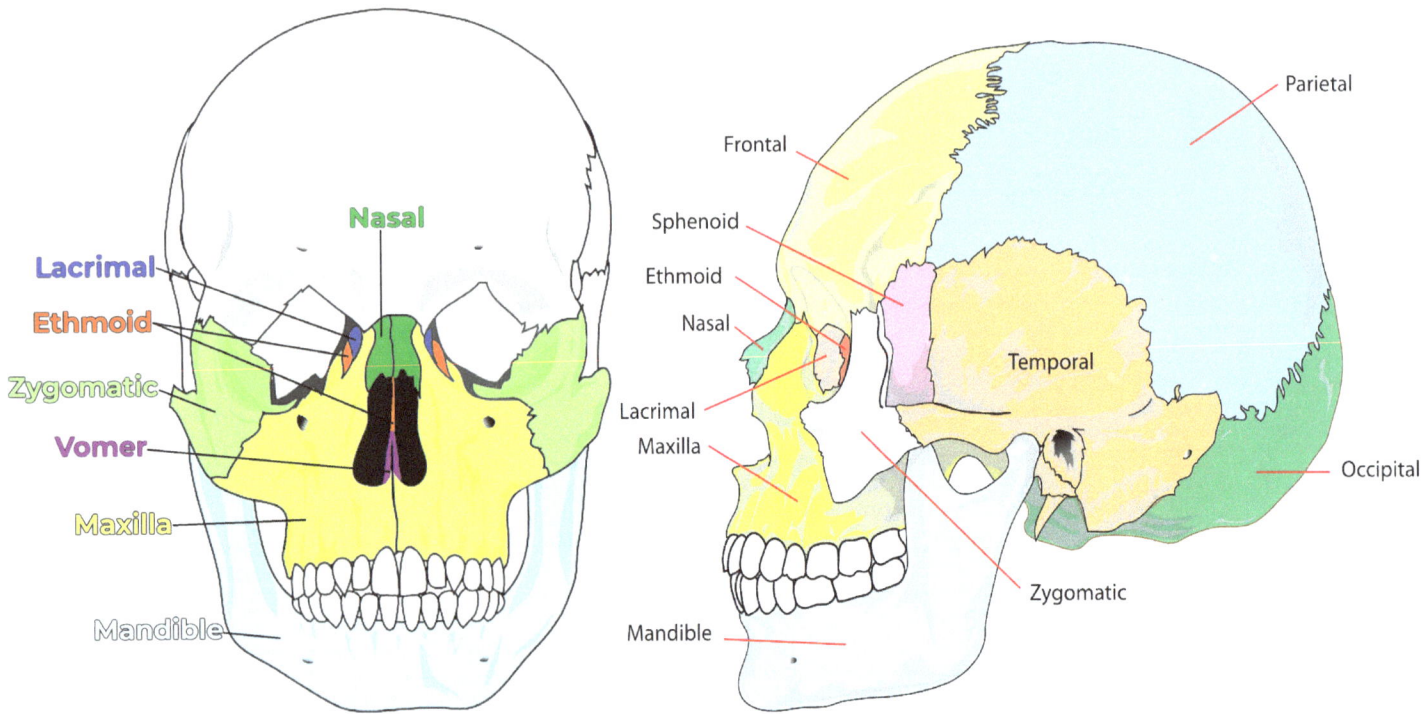

Nasal

Lacrimal

Ethmoid

Zygomatic

Vomer

Maxilla

Mandible

Frontal

Sphenoid

Ethmoid

Nasal

Lacrimal

Maxilla

Parietal

Temporal

Occipital

Zygomatic

Mandible

59 Bones of the face

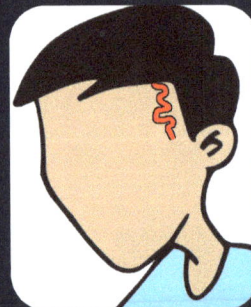

Sphenoid

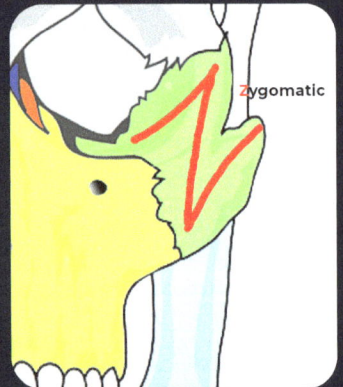

Zygomatic

1. **Sphenoid**: your vein starts popping out here when you get **enoid** (annoyed)
2. **Lacrimal**: simply think of where your **lacrimal (tear) duct** is
3. **Nasal**: Hmm, I wonder why it's called the nasal bone....(hint hint: it makes up your nose)
4. **Zygomatic**: looks like a "**Z**"
5. **Vomer**: looks like a **V** within a **V**
6. **Max**illa and **Mandible**: the two "ma-" bones make up most of the face, with the maxilla having more **maximal** height (i.e. the superior of the two)

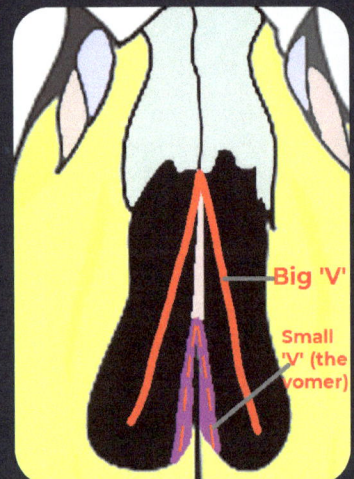

Big 'V'

Small 'V' (the vomer)

Vomer

CHAPTER 7

Arteries & Veins

60 Blood vessel terminology

Branch vs. tributary

Describes the **VESSEL**

Branch: splitting off of an artery
- Fairly obvious (if not, just think of how a tree branches out!)

Tributary: joining of a vein
- Remember the root word "**tribute**" or "con**tribute**" (i.e. the vein *contributes* to a larger vein)

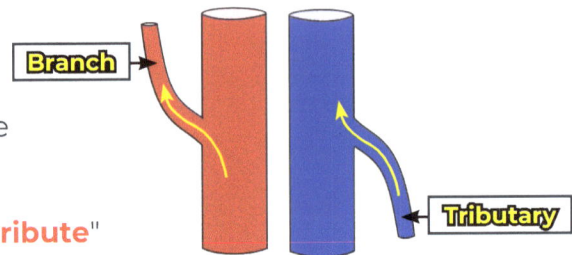

Anastomosis vs. bifurcation

Describes the **LOCATION**

Anastomosis: the spot where 2 blood vessels join
- Doesn't have to be 2 veins (i.e. can be used as a surgical term when you join any 2 structures)

Bifurcation: the spot where an artery divides into 2
- Either think about the word "bi-" which tells you it divides into two, or about "-**furc-**" which tells you it's a **fork** (e.g. *"fork in the road"*)

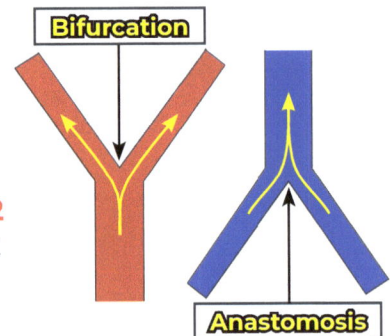

61 Blood vessel morphology terms

Some blood vessels are named according to the shapes they form or the directions they travel.

Circumflex = forms a circle

Circumflex arteries are *circular* arteries that wrap around something. The main ones are found in the upper and lower extremities and in the heart. In the arm, they wrap around the **humerus**; in the leg, around the **femur**; in the **heart**, around the...well, heart.

Profunda = profoundly deep

The word "profound" can mean "deep". Similarly, *profunda* arteries are branches of an artery that penetrate *deep* into a structure. The two major profunda to know are the **profunda femoris artery** in the **leg** and the **profunda brachii artery** in the **arm**. Note: sometimes these areteries are simply called *"deep"* instead of *profunda*.

Arcuate = forms an arch

Arcuate vessels or *"arches"* are literally *arch-shaped vessels* that join two larger vessels. The 3 main arches/arcuate vessels to know are in the 1. **hand** (palmar arches), 2. **foot** (arcuate artery and plantar arch), and 3. **kidney** (arcuate arteries & veins).

62 Basic artery pathways of extremities

> **Learn the main skeleton first, then STOP.
> Then slowly add in branches.**

The main arterial pathways, or "skeletons", of the upper and lower extremities are very simple. Learn these skeletons first before learning extensive branches, as they will confuse you when starting out. Get the most simple mental image of the path first, let it digest, and then add details as you go on.

Upper extremity

Every major arterial segment of the upper extremity is named according to what *area* it is located in. Therefore, think about the location and the names will come to you.

The **subclavian** artery is just **below** the **clavicle**; when it enters the **axilla** (armpit), it becomes the **axillary** artery; when it passes into the **arm**, it becomes the **brachial** artery (*brachial* means *'arm'*); it then splits off into two, following the forearm bones - one follows the **radius** (**radial** artery) and one follows the **ulna** (**ulnar** artery). The two of them then form 2 **arches** in the **palm** (**deep** and **superficial palmar arches**) through which they anastomose.

> ! Remember: on the right, the subclavian artery comes off the ***brachiocephalic trunk***, while on the left it comes *directly off the aorta* (there is no brachiocephalic trunk on the left!). This is different from the VENOUS system, where there *IS* both a right and left brachiocephalic vein!

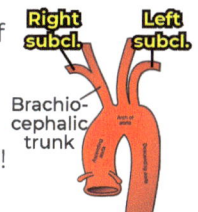

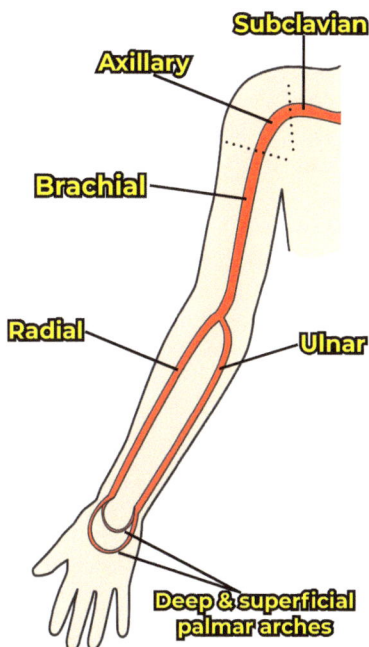

Labels (upper limb diagram): Subclavian, Axillary, Brachial, Radial, Ulnar, Deep & superficial palmar arches

Labels (aorta diagram): Right subcl., Left subcl., Brachiocephalic trunk

Lower extremity

The aorta bifurcates into the **common iliac arteries**. The fact that there's a *"common"* iliac artery tells you it must divide into two smaller iliac arteries - and it does, as the **internal** and **external iliac arteries**. The **internal** (also called the *hypogastric artery*) goes to the **internal** organs of the pelvis (reproductive organs, bladder, rectum, and more). The **external** goes to the **ex**tremity.

After crossing the **inguinal ligament**, the external iliac is called the **common femoral artery**. Again, *"common"* means there must be 2 smaller femoral arteries - these are the **deep (profunda)** and **superficial femoral arteries**. The deep femoral dives **deep** into the muscles of the thigh and supplies them, while the superficial femoral continues down the leg. At the knee, it becomes called the **pop**liteal artery (think: *knees can pop*). In the lower leg, the arteries are named after the bones - 2 arteries for the tibia (as it's the bigger one) and 1 for the fibula. The ***anterior*** tibial becomes the ***dorsalis* pedis** (makes sense that an <u>anterior</u> artery becomes a <u>dorsal</u> artery) and the ***posterior*** tibial eventually becomes the ***plantar* arch** (again, posterior-plantar relationship makes sense).

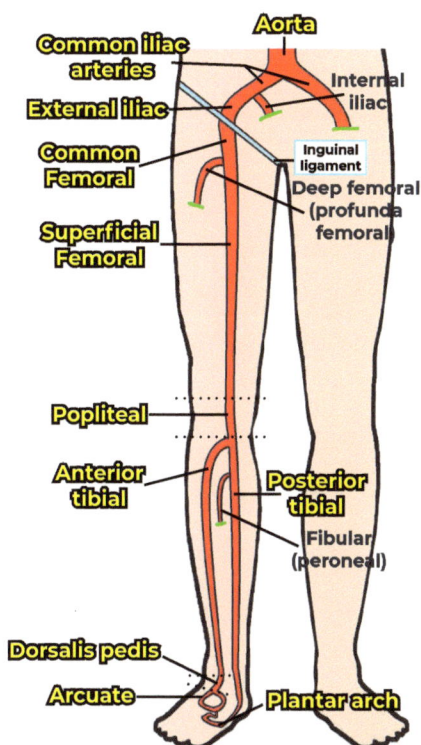

Labels (lower limb diagram): Common iliac arteries, Aorta, Internal iliac, External iliac, Common Femoral, Inguinal ligament, Deep femoral (profunda femoral), Superficial Femoral, Popliteal, Anterior tibial, Posterior tibial, Fibular (peroneal), Dorsalis pedis, Arcuate, Plantar arch

57

63 Bifurcation of the abdominal aorta

The abdominal aorta BiFOURcates at L4

Two easy ways to approximate the level of the L4 vertebra are to use the **iliac crest** or the **belly button** as landmarks (both are roughly at L4).

Similarly, remember that the **carotid artery** biFOURcates at **C4**!

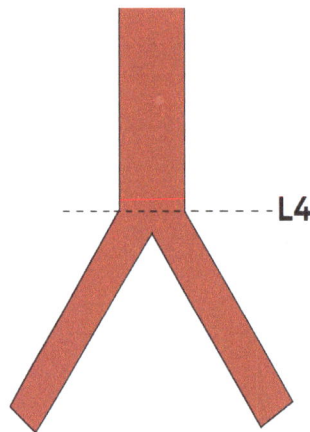

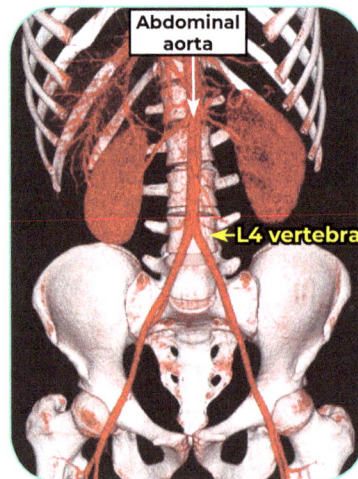

Abdominal aorta

L4

←L4 vertebra

! **Abdominal aortic aneurysm (AAA):** An AAA is when a portion of the abdominal aorta balloons out to **>3cm** in diameter. This is caused by things that **weaken the aortic wall**, like **smoking** and **atherosclerosis**. The larger the aneurysm, the higher the chance of rupture (often *FATAL!*). If the aneurysm is too close to the aortic bifurcation, it can complicate the surgical treatment.

Aneurysm

Celiac — T12
SMA — L1
Renal arteries — L2
IMA — L3

64 Abdominal aorta branches

Remember the branches by centering everything around the <u>renal arteries.</u>

The **2 renal arteries** branch off at **L2.** The **superior mesenteric artery (SMA)** lies one level **superior** to it (**L1**), and the **inferior mesenteric artery (IMA)** lies one level **inferior** to it (**L3**).

Simply remember the **celiac artery** branching off at **T12** *separately*, as it does so at a *separate* vertebral region (thoracic as opposed to lumbar).

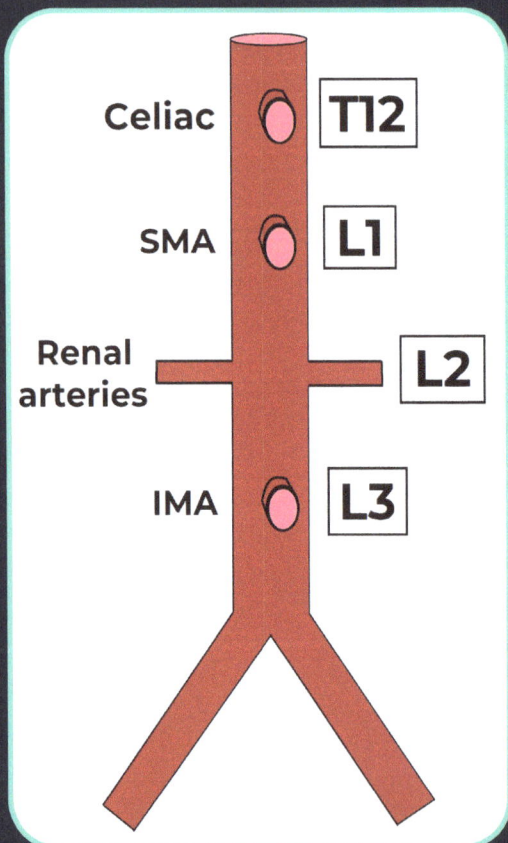

65 Celiac trunk branches

3 branches going to the 3 main organs in the area

The celiac trunk branches off into 3 arteries - each going to one of the major organs in the region (and hence being named after them:

1. **Splenic** artery (goes to **spleen**)
2. **Left gastric** artery (goes to **stomach**)
3. **Common hepatic** artery (goes to **liver**)

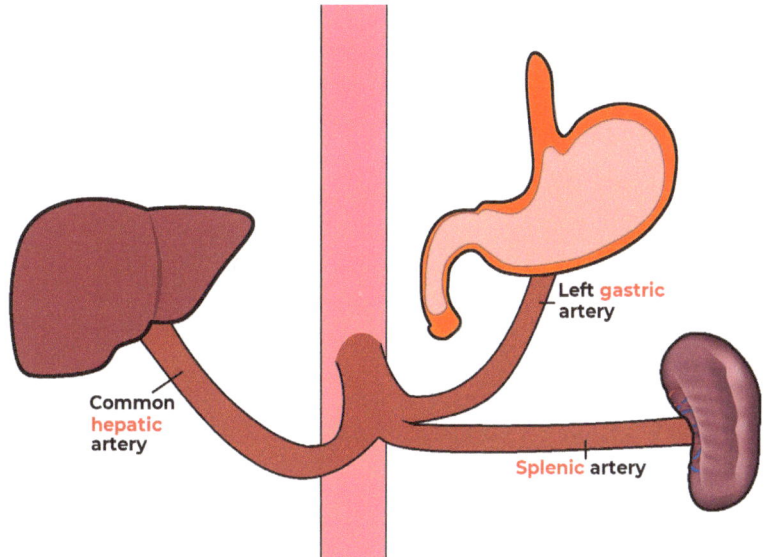

Left **gastric** artery

Common hepatic artery

Splenic artery

! Embryologically, the area supplied by the celiac trunk is known as the **FOREGUT**

66 SMA and IMA supply

Superior mesenteric artery (SMA): supplies **all of the intestines up until the left 1/3 of the transverse colon**

- **Duodenum, jejunum, ileum, ascending colon**, and **right 2/3 of the transverse colon**
- Embryologically, this entire region is called the **MIDGUT**
- The SMA also supplies the head of the pancreas

Inferior mesenteric artery (IMA): supplies **everything after SMA supply ends**

- **Left 1/3 of transverse colon, descending colon, sigmoid colon**, and **rectum** (upper 2/3)
- Embryologically, this entire region is called the **HINDGUT**

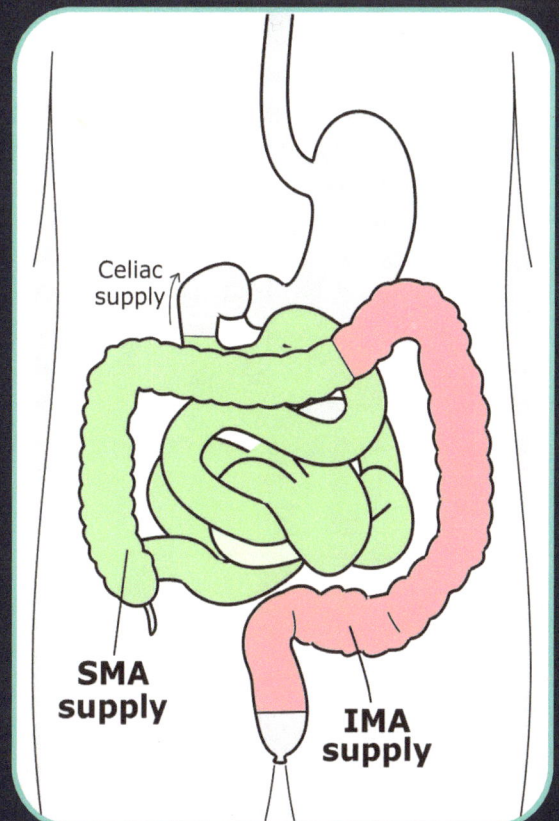

Celiac supply

SMA supply

IMA supply

67 Gonadal veins

"The Left gonadal vein takes the Longest way"

Venous drainage of the gonads:
- **Left** ovary/testis ➡ left gonadal vein ➡ *left renal vein* ➡ inferior vena cava (IVC)
- **Right** ovary/testis ➡ right gonadal vein ➡ IVC

Another intuitive way to think of it is to recall that the IVC is on the right side of the body, so naturally the left gonadal vein has to travel further to reach it.

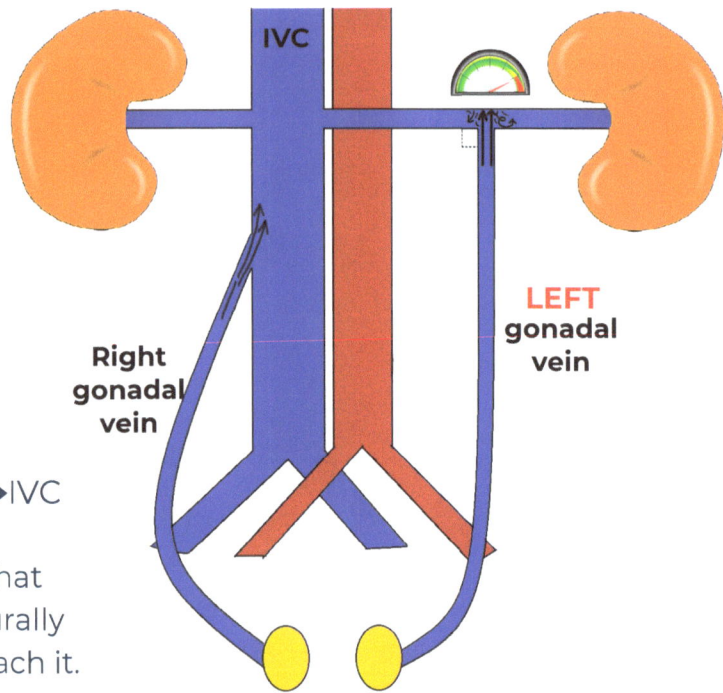

IVC

Right gonadal vein

LEFT gonadal vein

! **Importance**: Since the left gonadal vein enters the left renal vein at a ~90 degree angle, flow is less laminar on the left than on the right, leading to higher pressure on the left. This is why **varicocele** (swollen veins inside the scrotum) **is more common on the left**.

68 Uterine artery vs. ureter

Water (ureter) flows UNDER the bridge (uterine artery/vas deferens)

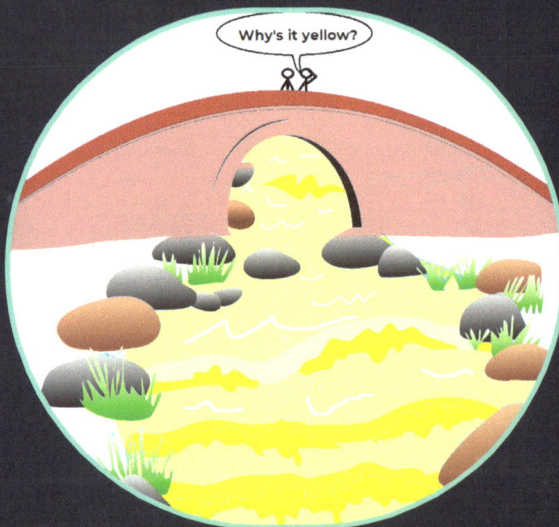

Why's it yellow?

The ureter passes **under** the uterine artery (or the vas deferens in males).

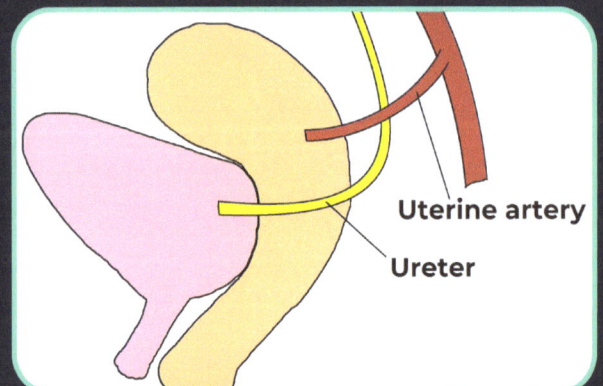

Uterine artery

Ureter

! **Importance**: This relationship is often tested because the ureter may be mistaken for the uterine artery during surgery and accidentally ligated, leading to an obstructed ureter.

Dr.You
METHOD

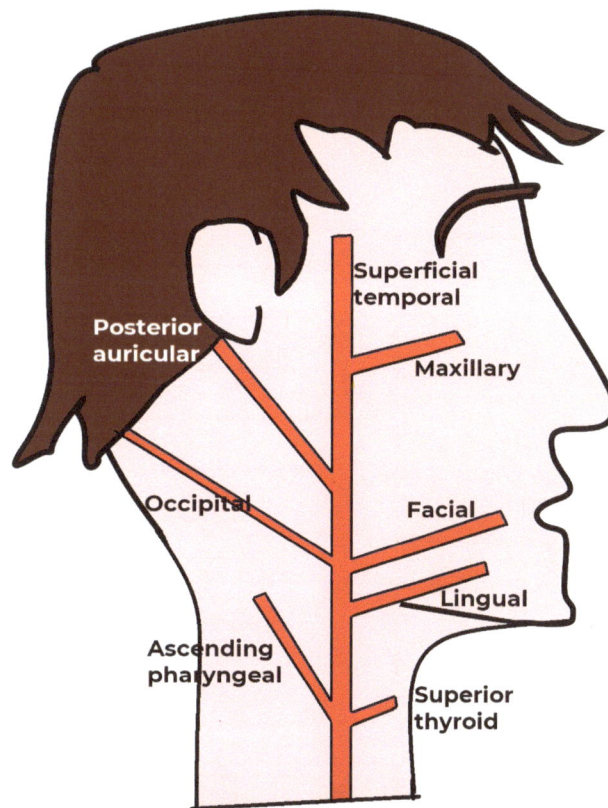

Superficial temporal

Posterior auricular

Maxillary

Occipital

Facial

Lingual

Ascending pharyngeal

Superior thyroid

69 External carotid artery branches

IN THE NAME!

SALFO-PMS

To make memorization of these branches immensely easier, remember that each branch is named after the structure it supplies, and that these structures start from the neck and progress superiorly. All you have to do is simply think about what structures you find as you work your way up your own neck and head:

8 branches, from inferior to superior:
- **S**uperior thyroid
- **A**scending pharyngeal
- **L**ingual
- **F**acial
- **O**ccipital
- **P**osterior auricular
- **M**axillary
- **S**uperficial temporal

- At the base of the neck lies your **thyroid** (hence your **superior thyroid** artery); above that you run into your **pharynx** (**ascending pharyngeal** artery), followed by your **tongue** (**lingual**), start of your **face** (**facial**), **occiput** (**occipital**), **ear** (**posterior auricular**), **maxilla** (**maxillary**), and **temple** (**superficial temporal**).

- To remember whether they travel anteriorly or posteriorly, again simply think about the structure they are supplying and their direction will be obvious.

61

NOTES

CHAPTER 8

Gastrointestinal

70 Omentum vs. mesentery

> **Mesentery = roots**
> **Omentum = apron**

Both mesentery and omentum are **folds of peritoneum** that **connect intraperitoneal organs** to something else. They are quite different however. Both their locations and functions can be understood by simply thinking of **mesentery as roots** and **omentum as an apron** (*omentum* literally means *apron*!).

Mesentery

Location: anchors **intraperitoneal organs** to the **posterior abdominal wall** (like roots)
- **Mes-entery** = *"**middle** of the **intestines**"* ("meso-" means *middle* [i.e. posterior wall], *"entero"* means *intestines*).

Function: **pathway for blood vessels, nerves, and lymphatics** from the abdominal wall to travel to the organs
- If you remember its attachment to the posterior wall, its function as a pathway for vessels, etc. makes perfect sense (the aorta and IVC are located BEHIND the peritoneal cavity, in the retroperitoneum).

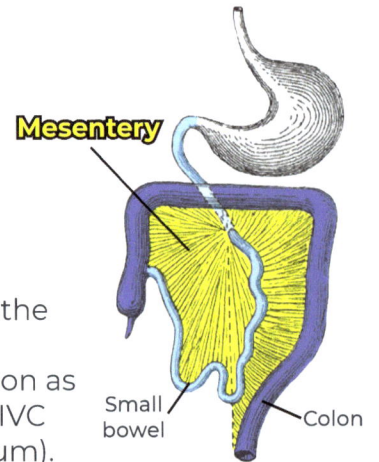

Omentum

Location: connects **STOMACH** to **other intraperitoneal organs.**
- *Greater* omentum: **stomach** to **transverse colon** (but hangs down like an apron)
- *Lesser* omentum: **stomach** to **liver**

Function: **"abdominal policeman"** (like an apron, it hangs in front of the abdominal organs and serves a protective/covering function).

1. **Infection/wound isolation:** omentum can actually physically wrap around areas of infection or trauma like a garment in order to isolate it and limit its spread.
2. **Immune:** has spots of macrophages that help fight off infection
3. **Fat deposition:** stores fat

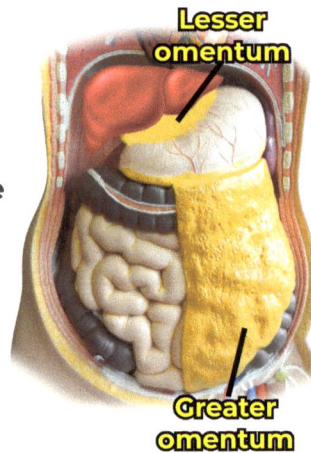

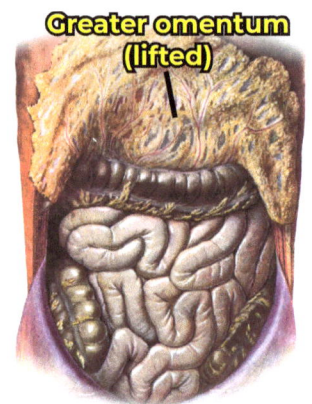

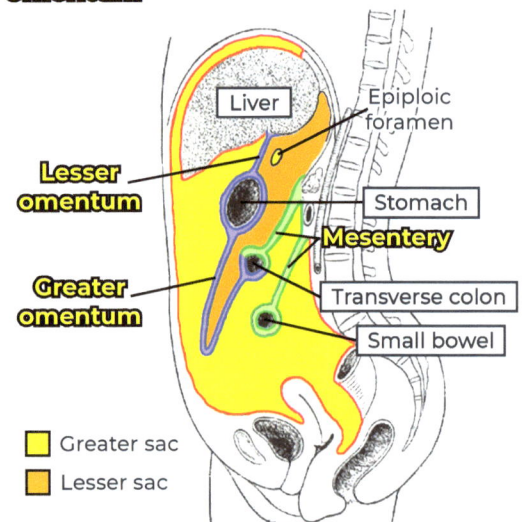

(!) **Greater and lesser sacs:** The peritoneal cavity is divided into two by the greater and lesser omenta: the **greater** and **lesser sacs**. There is a window in the lesser omentum that connects the two sacs called the **epiploic foramen (of Winslow)**. [Think: foramen of **Window**]

71

Retroperitoneal organs

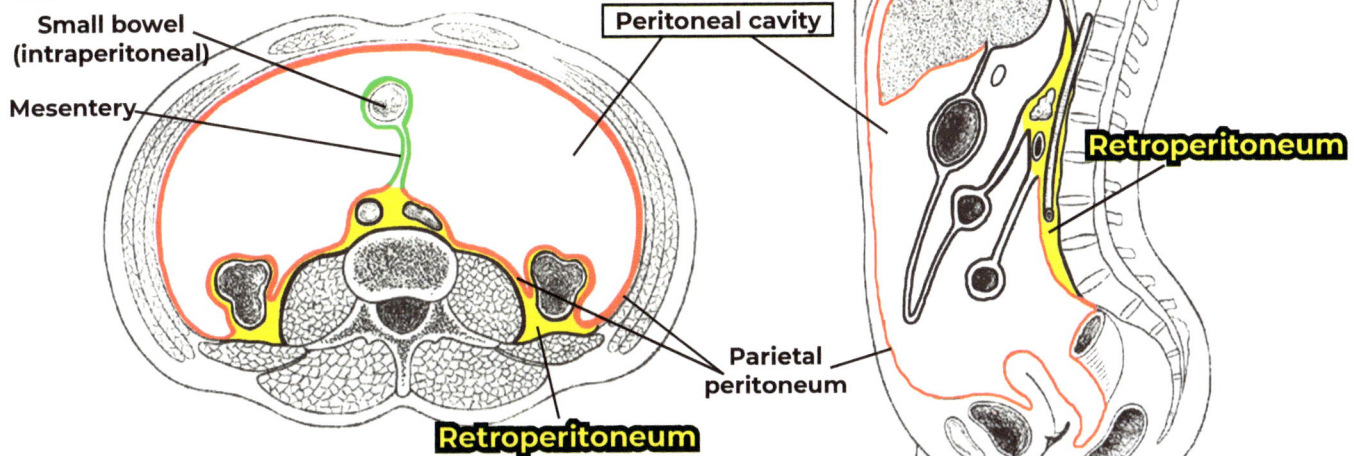

Small bowel
(intraperitoneal)

Mesentery

Peritoneal cavity

Retroperitoneum

Parietal
peritoneum

Retroperitoneum

Firstly, what is the retroperitoneum even?...

The retroperitoneum, as its name implies, is simply the space *behind* the *peritoneal cavity*. Think of the peritoneal cavity as the inside of a **bell pepper**, with the seeds representing organs suspended from the posterior abdominal wall. Retroperitoneal organs are more like **fruit stuck in jello**. Unlike the peritoneal cavity, which is essentially just a large potential space, the retroperitoneum is more tightly packed in and contains a lot of fascia and fat. It's not completely solid though, and there is still space in the retroperitoneum to bleed out into!

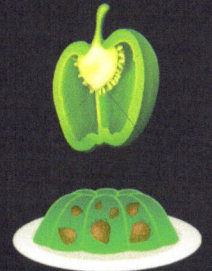

Note: Intraperitoneal organs are **suspended by mesentery**, while retroperitoneal organs are not.

Retroperitoneal organs

SADPUCKER

S: suprarenal (adrenal) gland
A: aorta/IVC
D: duodenum (2nd & 3rd part)
P: pancreas (except tail)
U: ureters
C: colon (ascending & descending)
K: kidneys
E: esophagus
R: rectum

Supplement this mnemonic with logic:

- The **aorta** and **IVC** are extremely important organs and it's befitting that they're retroperitoneal (offers protection)

- Most people know that the **kidneys** are located towards their back – hence it obviously must be retroperitoneal. The **ureters** and **adrenal glands** are both directly attached to the kidneys, hence they obviously must be retroperitoneal as well. So group these 3 organs together in your mind.

- Given that the anus lies towards the back side of your body, it makes sense that the **rectum** does as well (hence retroperitoneal).

- For the 3 retroperitoneal organs where the entire organ is not retroperitoneal (**duodenum**, **pancreas**, and **colon**), remember that in all 3 cases the MAJORITY of the organ is retroperitoneal, while only a minority is peritoneal.

72 Gastrointestinal ligaments

It's all in the name

For all except the falciform ligament, their names tell you exact what two structures they connect:

a) **Hepatoduodenal ligament**
Connects: liver to duodenum
Contains: portal triad
- <u>longest name</u> of all GI ligaments, so befitting that it has the most stuff packed into it (portal triad)

b) **Splenorenal ligament**
Connects: Spleen to left kidney
Contains: splenic artery & vein
- only GI ligament that starts with "spleno-" so obviously it contains the splenic artery/vein...duh...

c) **Falciform ligament**
Connects: liver to anterior abdominal wall
Contains: ligamentum teres hepatis (round ligament of liver) - which is the remnant of the fetal umbilical vein
- think: the FALCiform ligament contains the FALSE vein

d) **Gastrocolic**
Connects: stomach (greater curvature) to transverse colon

e) **Gastrosplenic**
Connects: stomach (greater curvature) to spleen

f) **Gastrohepatic**
Connects: liver to stomach (lesser curvature); separates greater and lesser sacs (can be cut during surgery to access lesser sac)

73 Diaphragmatic apertures (openings)

I ate 10 eggs at 12

I (IVC) **ate** (8) **ten** (10) **eggs** (esophagus) **at** (aorta) **twelve** (12)

At the following levels, these structures pass through the diaphragm:

T8: IVC
T10: esophagus
T12: aorta

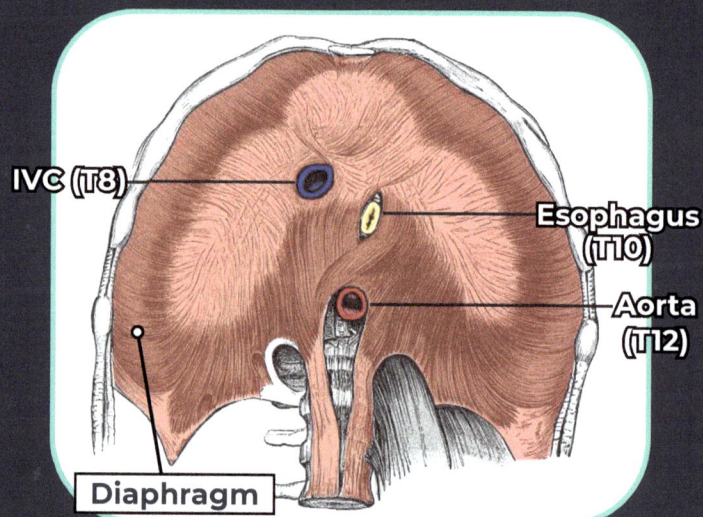

IVC (T8)
Esophagus (T10)
Aorta (T12)
Diaphragm

74 Small vs. large bowel folds

Small bowel

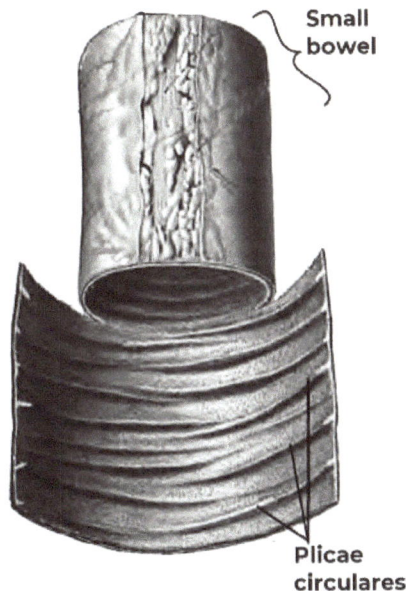

Small bowel

Plicae circulares

Large bowel

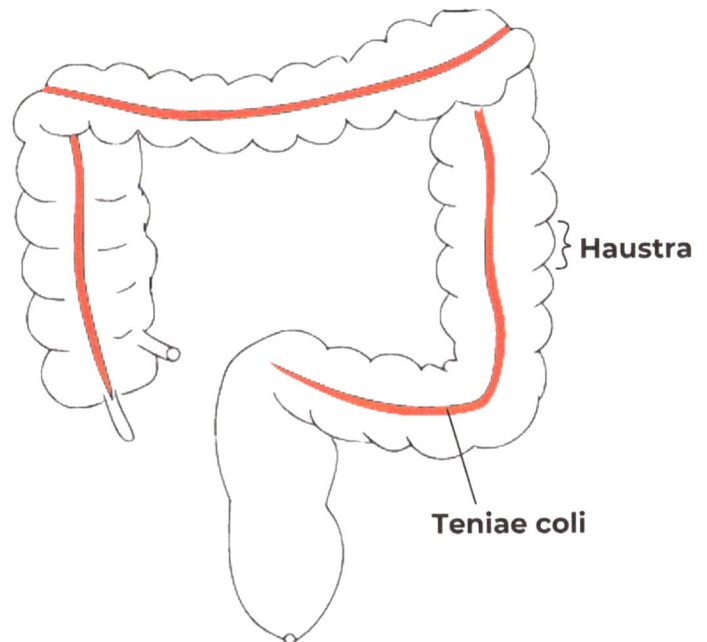

Haustra

Teniae coli

The small bowel has puny plicae circulares.

The large bowel has huge haustra.

Plicae circulares (also called *valvulae* or *circular folds*) are folds found in the small bowel. They are more numerus and are closer together (*"puny"*) than haustra. They function to increase the surface area of the small bowel for absorption.

Haustra are the **huge** pouches found throughout the large bowel (colon). They are less numerous and are wider apart than plicae circulares (think: everything is **larger** in the **large** intestines). They are formed by the lengthwise contraction of the *teniae coli* - the ribbon-like smooth muscle along the colon.

(!) **Importance**: These differences help in distinguishing between the small intestines and colon on abdominal x-ray and other imaging modalities.

Small bowel

Plicae circulares

Small bowel on X-ray

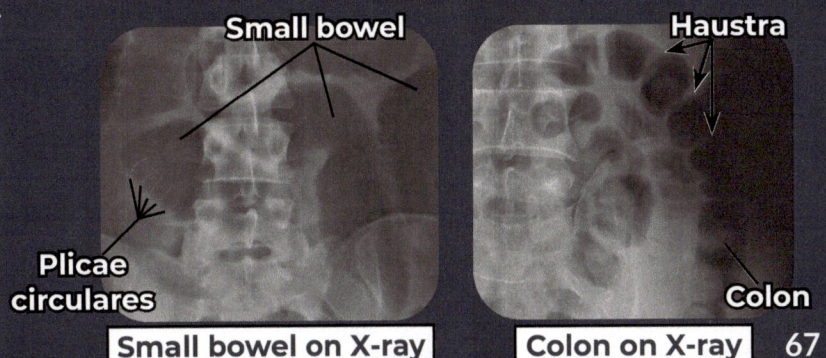

Haustra

Colon

Colon on X-ray

75 Layers of the abdominal wall

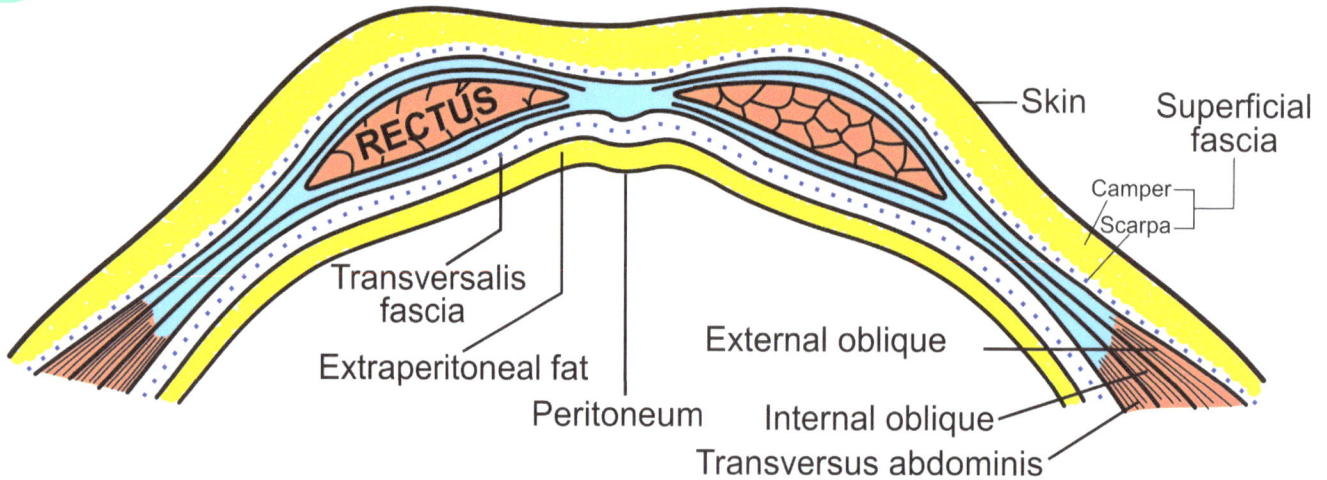

Labels: Skin · Superficial fascia · Camper · Scarpa · RECTUS · Transversalis fascia · Extraperitoneal fat · Peritoneum · External oblique · Internal oblique · Transversus abdominis

Muscle sandwich (almost perfectly symmetrical)

Muscles lie at the center of the abdominal wall. On either side of them is **fascia**, followed by **fat**, then a **final thin layer** (**skin** on outside, **peritoneum** on inside).

Thin layer → 1. **Skin**
Fat → 2. **Camper fascia** (really just **fat**)
Fascia → 3. **Scarpa fascia**
Muscles → 4. **Muscles**
  • **External oblique**
  • **Internal oblique**
  • **Transversus abdominis**
Fascia → 5. **Transversalis fascia**
Fat → 6. **Extraperitoneal fat**
Thin layer → 7. **Parietal peritoneum**

*Remember to use names to help you! (e.g. extra-peritoneal fat lies just outside the peritoneum, the external oblique muscle is outside the internal oblique, etc.)

- Remember that **Camper fascia** is *superficial* to **Scarpa fascia** by either remembering they follow **alphabetical order (C** before **S)** or that you go **camping** *outside*.
- Fascia functions to keep things like muscles and vessels in place, hence it makes sense that there is fascia immediately above and below the layer of muscles!

(!) <u>**Rectus** **sheath:**</u> In the more lateral parts of the abdominal wall, the external oblique, internal oblique, and transversus abdominis exist as actual muscles. More medially though, they become aponeuroses (broad, flat tendons) and cover the **rectus** abdominis (the "abs" or "6 pack") and **pyramidalis** muscles - hence the name *rectus* sheath! How many of the 3 aponeuroses that pass *in front* of the rectus abdominis changes at the **arcuate line** (a point about midway between the pubic symphysis and umbilicus):
  - **BELOW arcuate line:** all 3 aponeuroses pass in front
  - **ABOVE arcuate line:** 1.5 aponeuroses pass in front (external oblique + half of internal oblique) while 1.5 pass behind (*seen in image above*)

76   Hernias

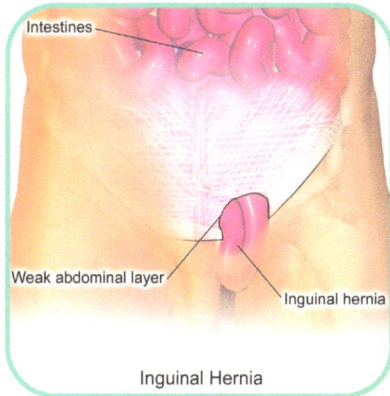

Intestines

Weak abdominal layer

Inguinal hernia

Inguinal Hernia

Indirect inguinal hernia

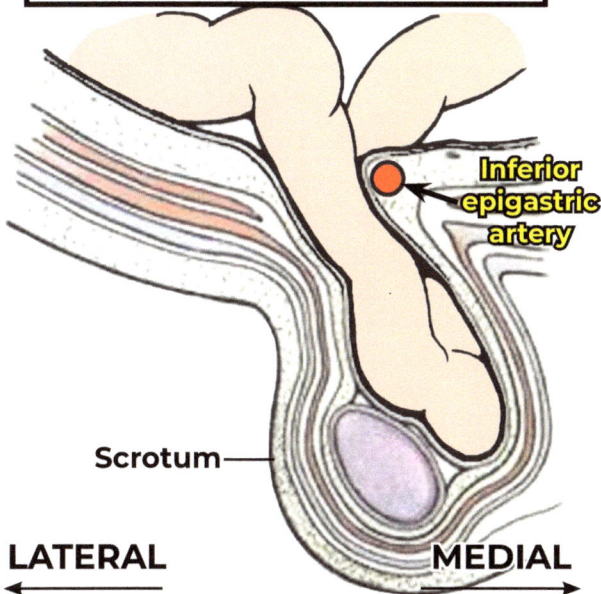

Inferior epigastric artery

Scrotum

LATERAL ⟵   MEDIAL

Direct inguinal hernia

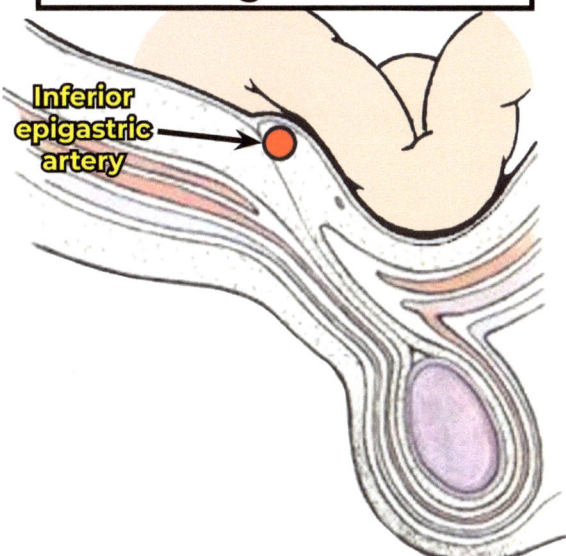

Inferior epigastric artery

- **INdirect inguinal hernias pass INto the inguinal canal** (while direct inguinal hernias poke through the abdominal wall).
- **FEMoral hernias are more common in FEMales.**

INdirect inguinal hernias occur in **INfants** because the **processus vaginalis** (developmental outpouching of peritoneum) travels through the inguinal canal and into the scrotum during development. This **communication between the abdomen and scrotum** is supposed to close around birth, but if it doesn't, then you have an open communication the two, which is just begging for a hernia to squeeze through it!

Direct inguinal hernias occur in **older men** because they form due to an **acquired weakness in the abdominal wall** (transversalis fascia). Older men have weaker abdominal walls. The inguinal canal is not the issue here!

Remember that **indirect inguinal hernias pass lateral to the inferior epigastric artery** (vs. medial for direct hernias) because the inguinal canal travels from lateral to medial to reach the groin.

! Remember: femoral hernias occur more in females than in males, but the most common groin hernia in females is still indirect inguinal hernias!

69

77 Portal venous system

What is the portal venous system?

The portal venous system is simply the venous drainage system of abdominal organs where the blood **passes through the liver first** before going to the heart. Systemic venous drainage, on the other hand, goes straight to the heart. *MOST* abdominal organs have portal venous drainage.

What is the point of the portal system?

The point of venous blood stopping first at the liver is to 1. **detoxify food** and its metabolites before it goes to the rest of the body, including the brain, and 2. **store** carbohydrates and vitamins/minerals extracted from food.

What organs does it drain?

GI tract (distal esophagus to upper anal canal), **pancreas, gallbladder,** and **spleen.**
- Think: *all abdominal organs related to food + the spleen.*
- It makes sense that the spleen has portal drainage because the spleen filters dead/damaged red blood cells, the breakdown products of which require *processing.*

Abdominal organs that *DO NOT* have portal drainage: 1. kidneys, 2. liver itself.

What main veins are involved?

All **portal** venous drainage enters the liver through the **portal** vein. The portal vein is formed by the **S**uperior mesenteric vein and the **S**plenic vein (think: SS Port ['SS' like the ship prefix]). The **inferior mesenteric vein** drains into the splenic vein. Blood leaves the liver via the **hepatic vein.**
- The portal venous system corresponds roughly to areas supplied by the *celiac trunk, superior mesenteric artery,* and *inferior mesenteric artery.*

What are porto-systemic anastomoses?

Porto-systemic anastomoses are places where portal and systemic veins connect with each other. There are 3 major sites where this happens:
1. **Esophagus**
   - Between *left gastric* (portal) and *azygos* (systemic) veins
2. **Rectum**
   - Between *superior rectal* (portal) and *middle/inferior rectal* (systemic) veins
3. **Umbilicus**
   - Between *paraumbilical* (portal) and *small epigastric* (systemic) veins

Why does this all matter?

1. **Varices:** Pathology of the liver that causes obstruction to the portal system (e.g. cirrhosis, tumor, portal vein thrombosis) can increase the pressure in the portal system (*portal hypertension*). This can cause blood to back up into the porto-systemic anastomoses and cause them to dilate over time - called **varices.** Varices can rupture and lead to life-threatening hemorrhage.

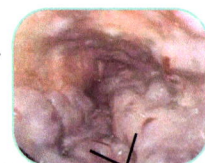
Esophageal varices

2. **Hepatic encephalopathy:** When the liver can't detoxify the portal blood well due to some liver disease, the toxins can go to the brain unfiltered, causing a decline in brain functioning.
3. **First-pass metabolism:** Some drugs aren't taken orally because the portal system takes them to the liver first ("*first*-pass metabolism"), which just inactivates them.

Dr.**You**
METHOD

Portal venous system

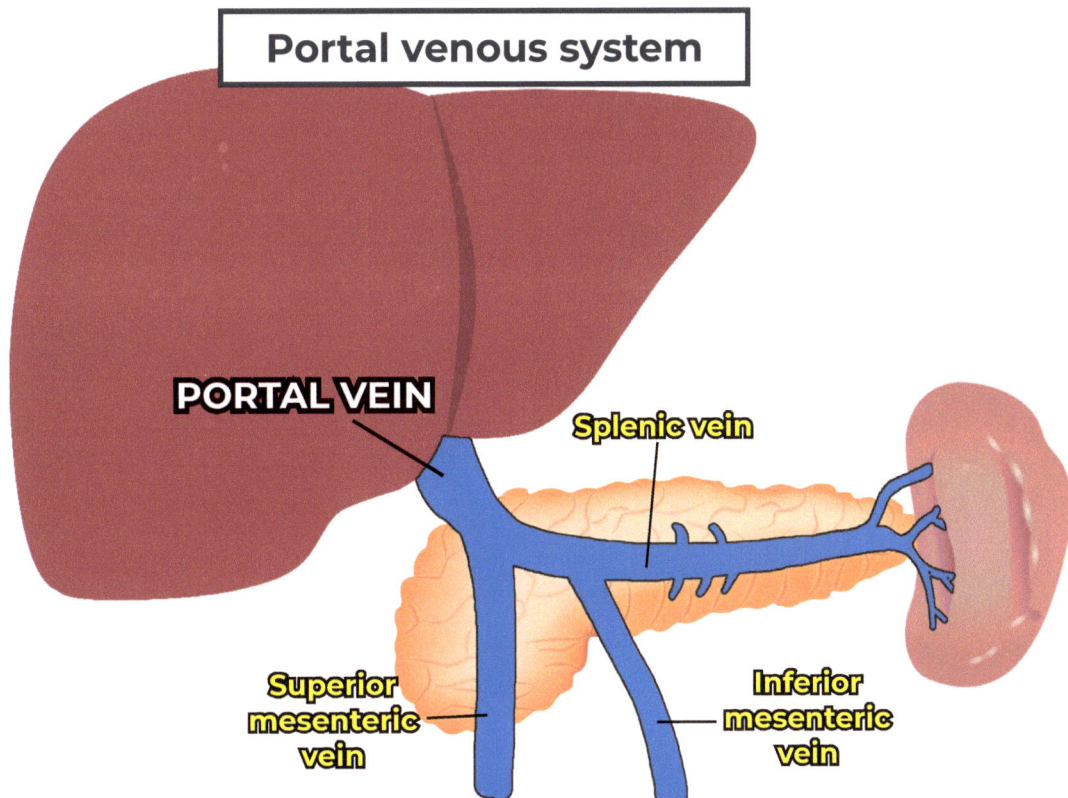

PORTAL VEIN

Splenic vein

Superior mesenteric vein

Inferior mesenteric vein

---

78 Median vs. medial umbilical ligaments

> **Median** = *"exactly in the midline"* = only **1** of it = urachus
> **Medial** = *"towards midline"* = must be **2** (1 on each side) = umbilical arteries

The median and medial umbilical ligaments are simply remnants of embryonic structures that have been obliterated and are now just ligaments attached to the umbilicus.

- The **median umbilical ligament** contains the **urachus**, which is a remnant of the canal that drains the **urinary bladder** of the fetus (the *allantois*). In the adult, it supports the bladder by attaching it to the umbilicus.
- The **medial umbilical ligaments** are remnants of the two **umbilical arteries**.

This can be easily remembered by understanding that:

- **Median** means "*in the midline*", which means there can be only **one** of it. It thus makes sense that it contains the urachus (fetus only has one urachus, just like we have only one urethra!)
- **Medial** just means "*towards the midline*", which tells you there must be **2** - one on each side of the midline. It thus makes sense that they correspond to the 2 umbilical arteries.

(!) Note: there are also the lateral **umbilical ligaments** - which contain the **inferior epigastric arteries**.

79 Liver segments

Anterior view

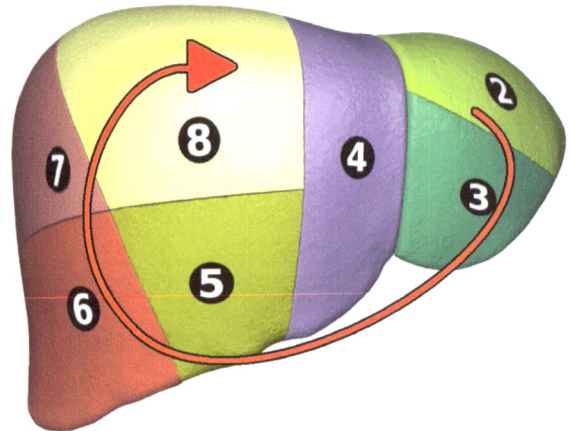

> Segments are numbered in a **clockwise fashion** (aside from segment 1)

To remember the numbering of the liver segments, count **segment 1 (caudate lobe)** as the outlier hiding at the back of the liver - then simply follow a **clockwise pattern**, starting from the liver's left edge.

This numbering system is based on the bifurcation of the main blood supply of the liver - the **portal vein**.

Posterior view

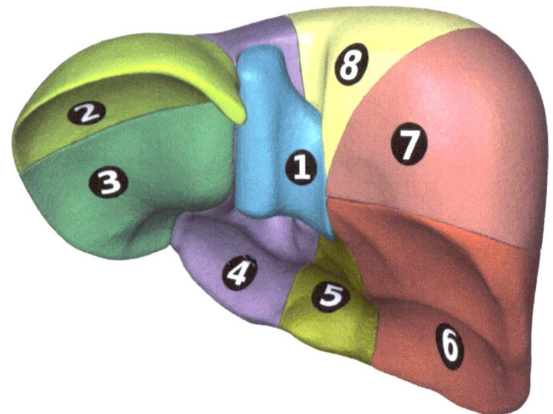

(!) Alternatively, the liver is often referred to as having **medial** and **lateral** segments, divided by the **ligamentum teres** (notice the indentation on the bottom edge of the liver between segments 3 and 4?)

80 Relation of the pancreas and spleen

> The tail of the pancreas *tickles* the spleen

The spleen is positioned at the tip of the tail of the pancreas, coming in direct contact with it.

(!) **Importance**: This is an important relation to remember because an inflamed pancreas (pancreatitis) can **spread its inflammation to the adjacent splenic vein**, causing **splenic vein thrombosis**.

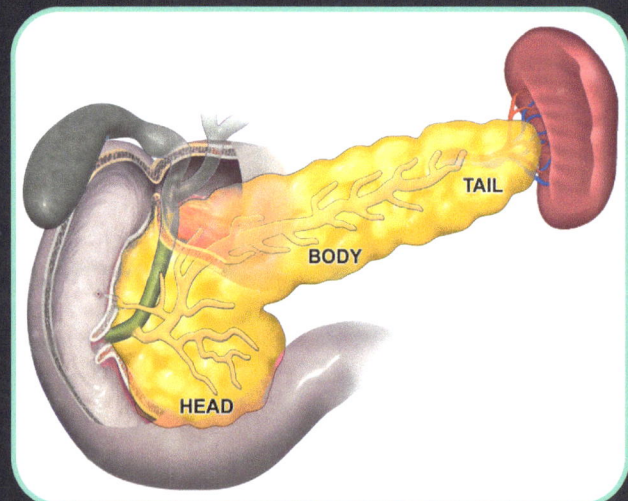

81 Most dependent parts of the abdomen

> **Pouch of Douglas: deepest hole that can be dug**
> **Hepatorenal recess: the liver being the biggest organ, it creates the deepest pouch**

The most dependent (i.e. lowest) placest in the peritoneal cavity (hence where fluid would accumulate if present) are:

- **When upright: rectouterine pouch (pouch of Douglas)**, located between the rectum and uterus (females only, of course)
- **When supine: hepatorenal recess (Morrison's pouch)**, located between the liver and right kidney.

(!) In trauma, blood can collect in these spots, and you can check for it using an ultrasound or CT scan.

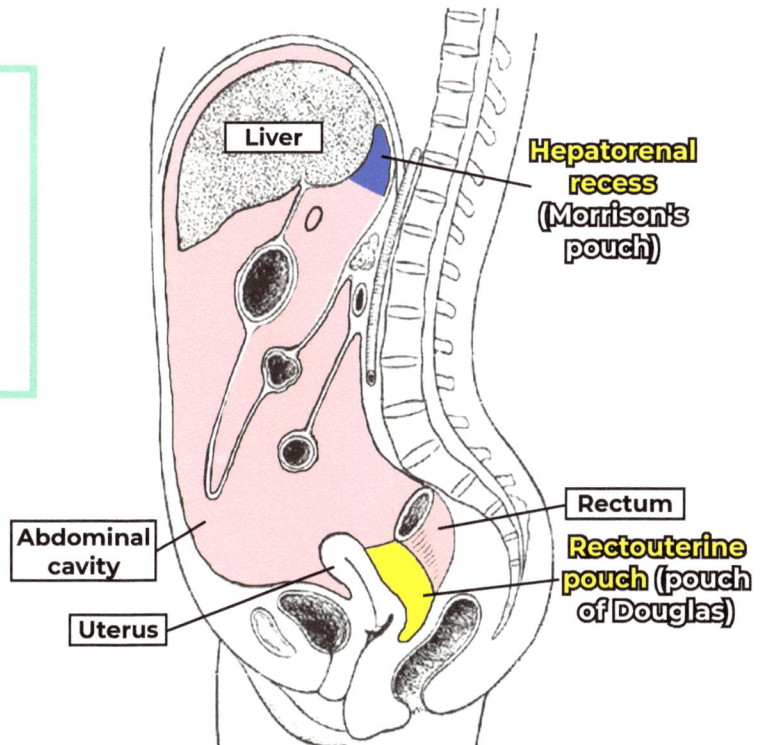

Liver · Hepatorenal recess (Morrison's pouch) · Abdominal cavity · Uterus · Rectum · Rectouterine pouch (pouch of Douglas)

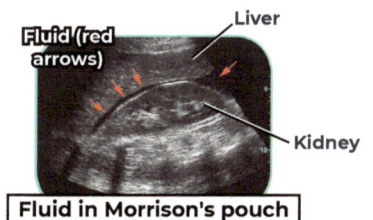

Fluid (red arrows) · Liver · Kidney

Fluid in Morrison's pouch

82 Production vs. storage of bile

> **The gallbladder only *stores* the bile, just like the urinary bladder only *stores* urine**

Liver: *produces* bile
Gallbladder: *stores* bile

Much like the urinary bladder only storing urine, the gallbladder simply stores the bile produced by the liver.

(!) In those who have had their gallbladder removed ("cholecystectomy"), which is often done in gallstone disease, their liver still secretes bile - they just can't store it!

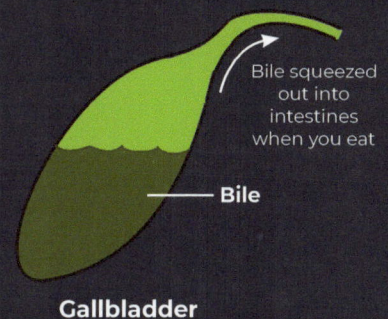

Bile squeezed out into intestines when you eat · Bile · Gallbladder

NOTES

CHAPTER 9

Cardiovascular

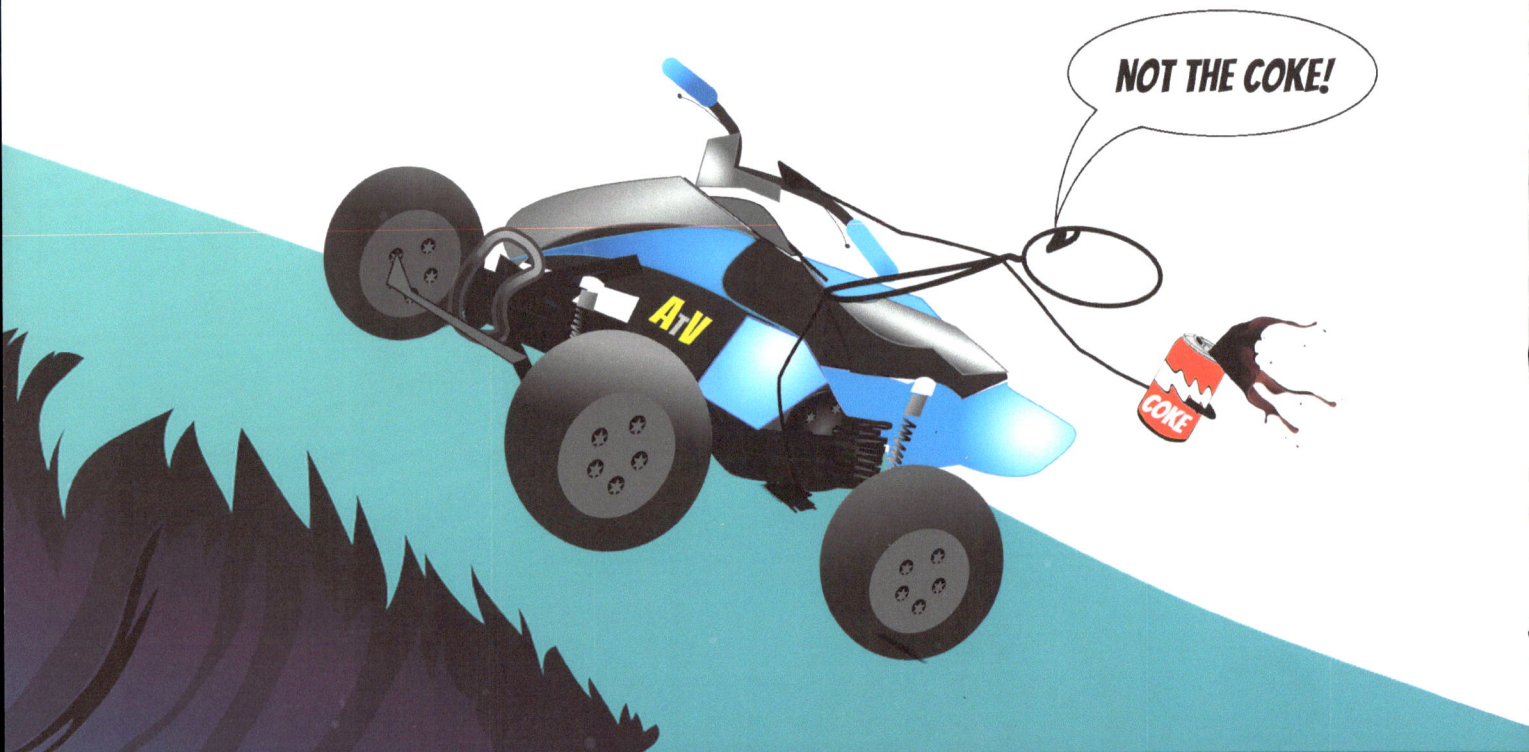

NOT THE COKE!

A͏V

COKE

83 Triangle of Koch

See the Coke being spilled on the AtV

The atrioventricular (AV) node is located in the triangle of Koch (literally pronounced "coke").

! **Importance**: The triangle of Koch serves as an important **anatomical landmark** for locating the AV node during procedures such as pacing or catheter ablation (destroying areas of heart tissue that are causing arrhythmia).

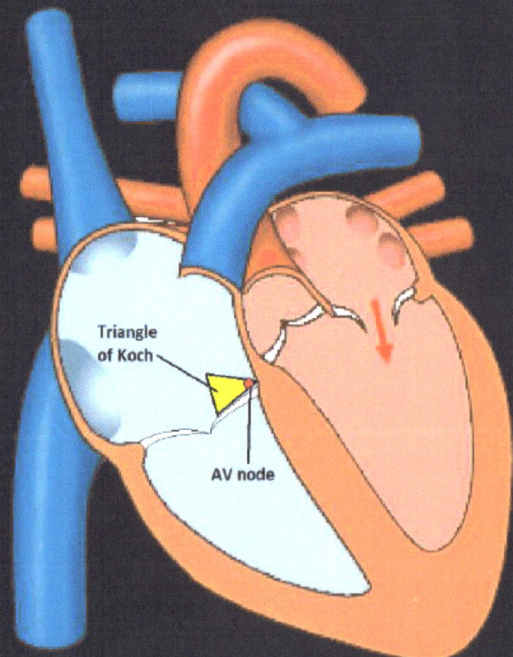

Triangle of Koch

AV node

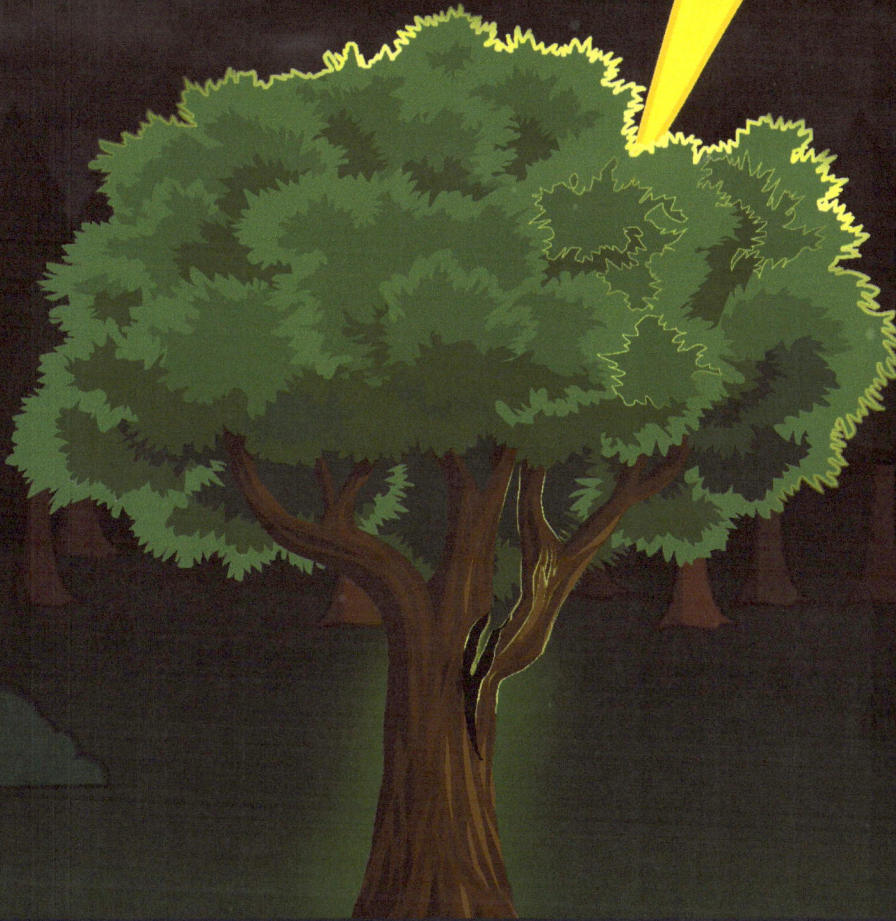

SAAV His Branch!!!

84 Cardiac conduction pathway

SAAV His Branch!

The conduction system of the heart carries electrical impulses along this pathway:

1. **SA node** (pacemaker)
2. **AV node**
3. **Bundle of His**
4. **Bundle branches** (left and right)

See that poor little branch dangling after it was struck by lightning? The **lightning** should remind you of the **conduction system**, and that concerned man crying for someone to "**SAAV (save) His Branch**" denotes the pathway impulses take.

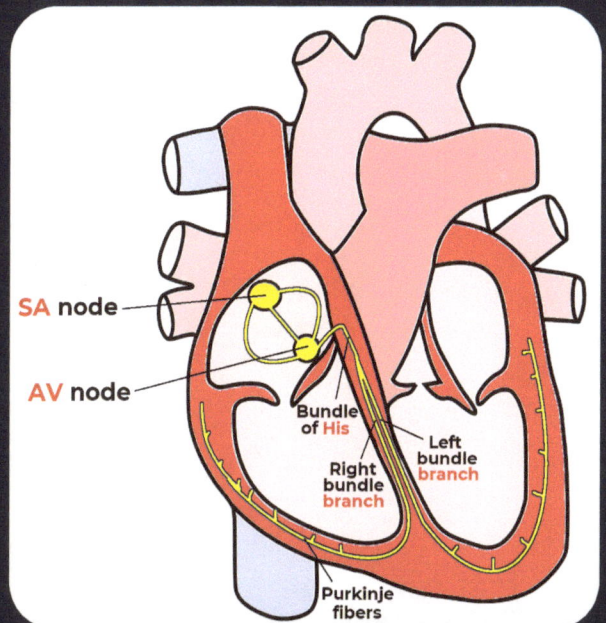

SA node

AV node

Bundle of His

Right bundle branch

Left bundle branch

Purkinje fibers

85 Posterior descending artery origin

> **Just as most people are right-handed, most people also have right-dominant circulation**

The **posterior descending artery** arises from the **right coronary artery** in ~85% of people (termed **right-dominant circulation**), while in a minority it arises from the **left circumflex artery** (**left-dominant circulation**).

86 Posterior-most heart chamber

> **The LA is the LAst part of the heart before the esophagus**

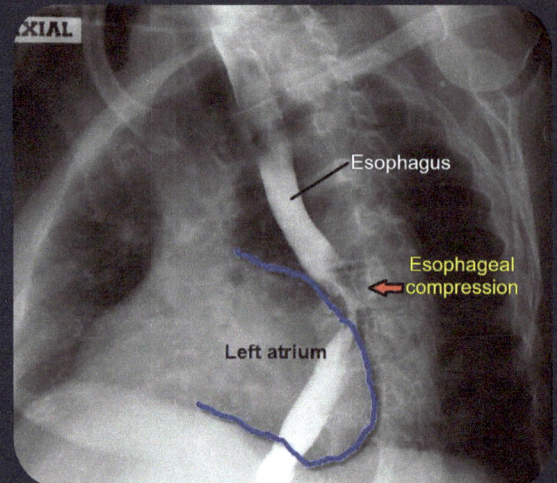

Esophagus

Esophageal compression

Left atrium

The **left atrium** (**LA**) is the most posterior chamber of the heart, directly behind which is the esophagus.

(!) **Importance**: An enlarged left atrium (as seen in mitral stenosis and heart failure, for example) may **externally compress the esophagus**, causing **dysphagia** (difficulty swallowing).

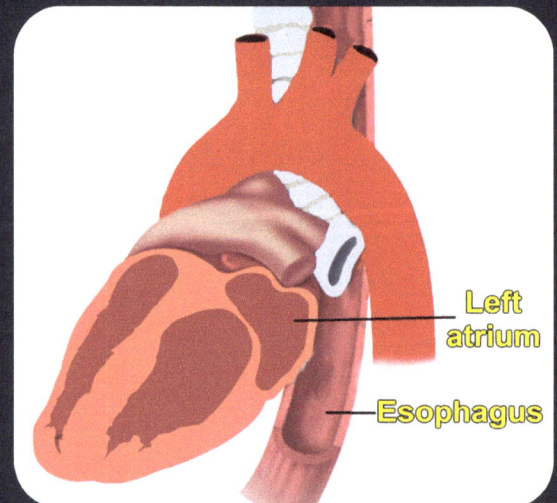

Left atrium

Esophagus

87 Tricuspid vs. mitral valve

> ## Exact same as lung lobes (3 on right, 2 on left)

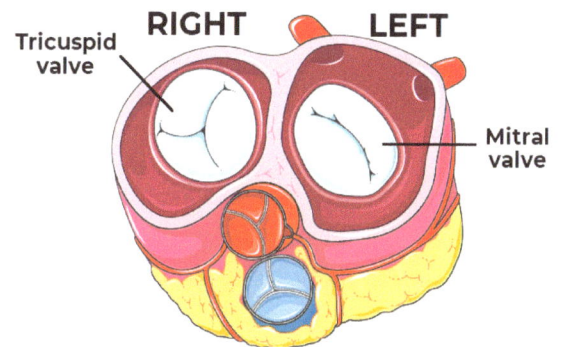

RIGHT LEFT

Tricuspid valve

Mitral valve

Between the atria and ventricles lie:

Right heart: Tricuspid valve (3 cusps)
Left heart: Mitral valve (2 cusps)

To remember which valve lies on which side, simply think of the **lungs** - the **number of lobes in each lung** exactly matches the **number of valve cusps on each side of the heart**!

88 Muscles of the heart's inner surface

The *myocardium* is the _actual wall_ of the heart. It's what actually pumps the blood. On the other hand, there are several muscles that are simply part of the _inner lining_ of the heart:

Pectinate muscles vs. trabeculae carneae

The walls of the atria and ventricles contain ridges of muscles. The **atria have pectinate muscles**, while the **ventricles have trabeculae carneae**.

- **Pectinate muscles (atria):** smooth appearance
- **Trabeculae carneae (ventricles):** irregular, sponge-like. *Papillary muscles* are one type of trabeculae carneae.
  - Trabeculae carneae means *"trabeculated (beam-like) meat"*
  - Think: *the atria are low pressured and hence their walls are soft and smooth, while the ventricles are a wild, wild place with high pressures and funky muscles*

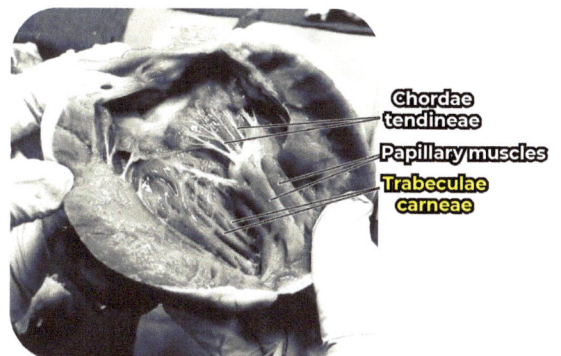

Chordae tendineae
Papillary muscles
Trabeculae carneae

Papillary muscles and chordae tendineae

Papillary muscles are the muscles coming off the walls of the ventricles that **pull on the mitral and tricuspid valves** to **prevent them from inverting or prolapsing** during systole. They do so via the **chordae tendineae** (sometimes called *"heart strings"*), which as the name implies, are simply the **cords** between the papillary muscles and the heart valves.

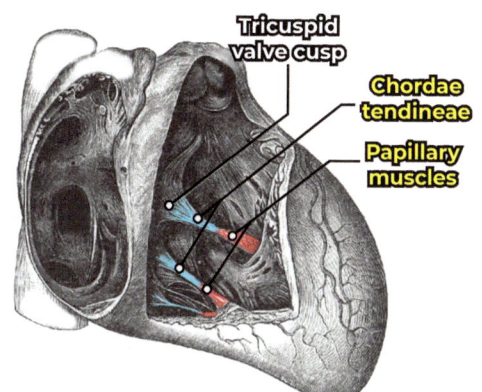

Tricuspid valve cusp
Chordae tendineae
Papillary muscles

NOTES

CHAPTER 10

Endocrine

89   Adrenal cortex: layers & hormones

a) Layers

GFR

From superficial to deep:

- Zona **G**lomerulosa
- Zona **F**asciculata
- Zona **R**eticularis

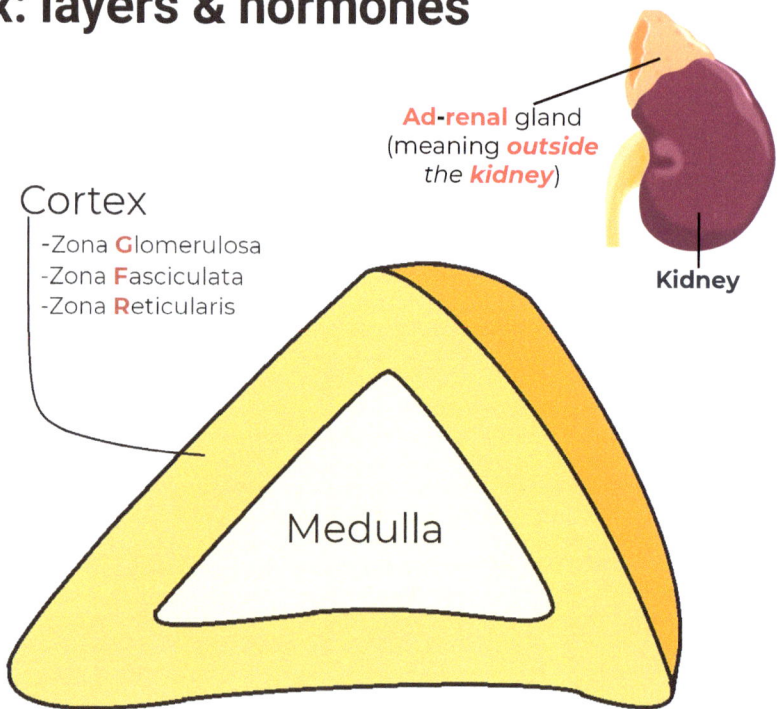

Cortex
- Zona **G**lomerulosa
- Zona **F**asciculata
- Zona **R**eticularis

Ad-renal gland (meaning *outside the kidney*)

Kidney

Medulla

(Think GFR like *glomerular filtration rate*)

b) Hormones

"The **deeper** you go, the **sweeter** it gets!"

Hormone production, by layer, from superficial to deep:
- **Zona Glomerulosa: Salt (mineralocorticoids** i.e. aldosterone**)**
- **Zona Fasciculata: Sugar (glucocorticoids)**
- **Zona Reticularis: Sex (androgens)**

(!) **Adrenaline** (epinephrine) and **nor**adrenaline (norepinephrine) are produced at the very *core* of the adrenal gland - the **adrenal medulla**.

90 Pituitary gland and hormones

FLAT PiG

The anterior pituitary produces:
FSH (follicle-stimulating hormone)
LH (luteinizing hormone)
ATCH (adrenocorticotropic hormone)
TSH (thyroid-stimulating hormone)
Prolactin
(**i**gnore)
GH (growth hormone)

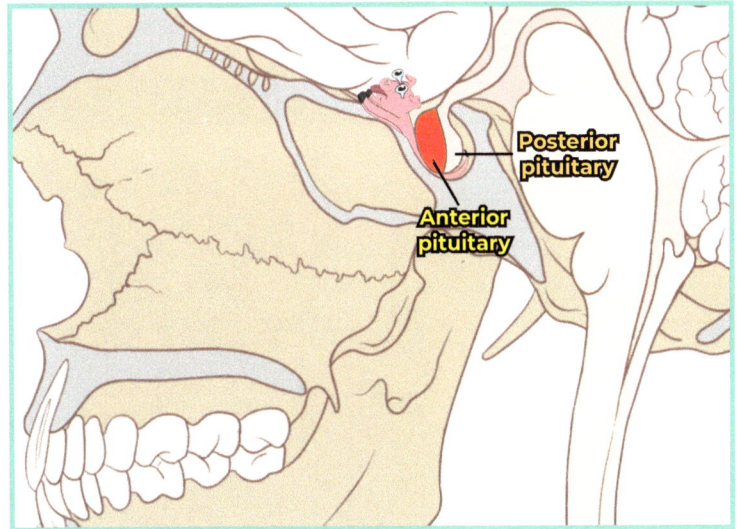

The posterior pituitary secretes only **oxytocin** and **anti-diuretic hormone** (*ADH*, also called *vasopressin*).

Remember: the anterior pituitary produces its **own hormones**, while the posterior pituitary simply secretes hormones that were **already produced by the hypothalamus**. It thus makes sense that the posterior pituitary is physically connected to the hypothalamus by a **stalk** (the anterior pituitary is *NOT*)! Think: the anterior pituitary is at the front because it's the *alpha-male* - it's bold, autonomous, and produces its own hormones - while the posterior pituitary is *passive* and is dependent on the hypothalamus.

91 Pineal gland

Pineal gland: makes you hit the pillow. Pea-shaped.

The pineal gland secretes **melatonin**, which regulates your sleep pattern. It is **pea-shaped** and it hangs right above the cerebellum ("**p**okes the cerebellum").

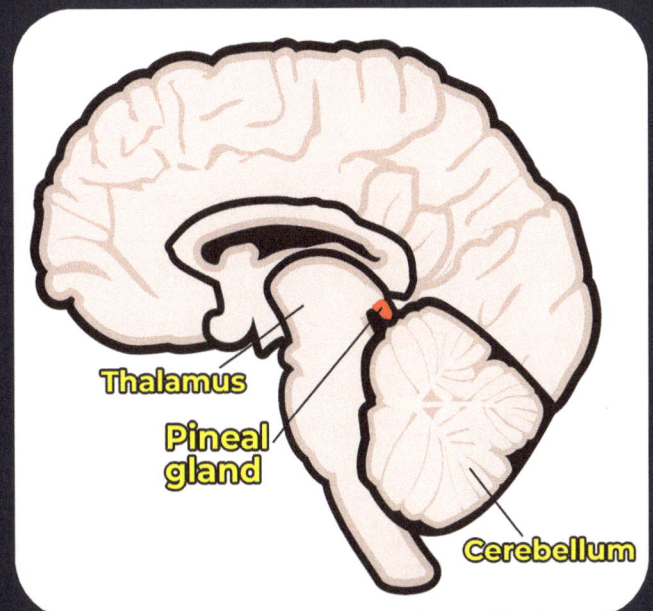

(!) **BONUS**: The word '**pine**al' is actually derived from '**pine-cone**', in reference to its cone shape.

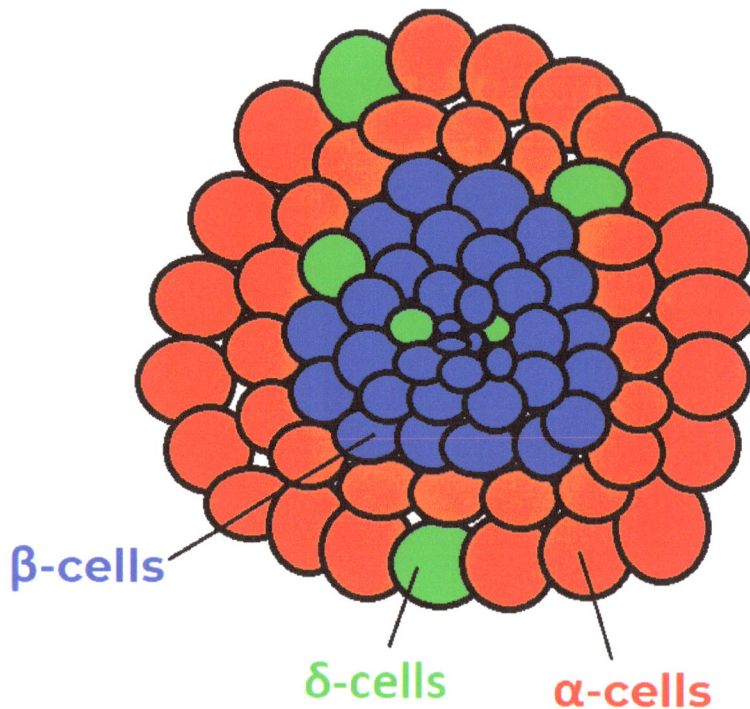

β-cells

δ-cells   **α-cells**

92

Endocrine pancreas: cell types & locations

> **α-cells: alpha males**
> **β-cells: Beta males**
> **δ–cells: no one cares about these**

The endocrine pancreas has clusters of cells called **islets of Langerhans**, which contain **α, β, and δ cells**. These cells are arranged within the islets in a particular pattern:

- **α-cells:** along the exterior edges because **alpha cells**, like **alpha** males, are extroverted and outgoing. They secrete **glucagon**.
- **β-cells:** hidden within the core because **Beta cells**, like **Beta males**, are shy. They secrete **insulin**. (Alternative: **Insulin** [B-cells] **inside**)
- **δ–cells:** think "no one really cares about these, so they don't even have a set location" **(interspersed;** secrete **somatostatin** [think: the symbol δ looks like an **'s'**])

CHAPTER 11

Hematology

93 Maturation of lymphocytes

> ## B cells mature in the bone marrow.
> ## T cells mature in the thymus.

(!) Remember that this mnemonic refers to the site of cell **MATURATION** – not production! Both B cells and T cells originate from stem cells in the **bone marrow**.

94 Granulocytes

BEN

Picture a guy named **Ben** with a ton of **granulated** acne.

A granulocyte is simply any white blood cell that has visible granules when stained. There are 3 granulocytes:

- **B**asophils
- **E**osinophils
- **N**eutrophils

Granules contain **toxins for killing pathogens** (e.g. nitric oxide, hydrogen peroxide, enzymes like lysozyme) or **mediators for inflammation** (e.g. in infections, asthma, allergic reactions) like histamine.

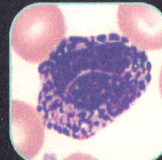

Basophil
Look for:
- Deeply purple
- PACKED with granules

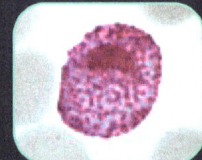

Eosinophil
Look for:
- Deeply pink
- Packed with granules

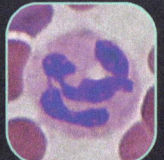

Neutrophil
Look for:
- Segmented nucleus

Naming: Granulocytes are named based on how they stain. Basophils stain basophilic (purple), eosinophils stain eosinophilic (pink), and neutrophils stain neutral (somewhere in between).

Neutrophil segments:
- 3-5 segments → Normal mature neutrophils
- < 3 segments → Bands (immature neutrophils)
- > 5 segments → Megaloblastic anemia

95 White blood cell differential count

> ## Reverse alphabetical order (*almost*)

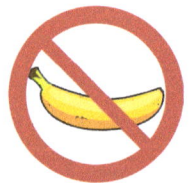

Under NORMAL conditions, the WBC differential count is, from highest to lowest:

Neutrophils (~60%)
Lymphocytes (~30%)
Monocytes (~6%)
Eosinophils (~3%)
Basophils (~1%)

(A) Alternative mnemonic:
"**N**ever **L**et **M**onkeys **E**at **B**ananas"

Alterations from the norm: Certain infections characteristically increase a certain type of WBC more than the others:
- **Bacteria:** neutrophils
- **Viruses:** lymphocytes
- **Fungi:** lymphocytes
- **Parasites:** eosinophils

96 Spleen location

> ## If you get hit in the spleen, call 9-1-1!

The spleen is located in the upper left abdomen at the level of ribs 9 to 11.

(!) The normal location and size of the spleen is important to know in order to detect **splenomegaly** (enlarged spleen), which is seen in many conditions, including certain anemias, malaria, and tumors.

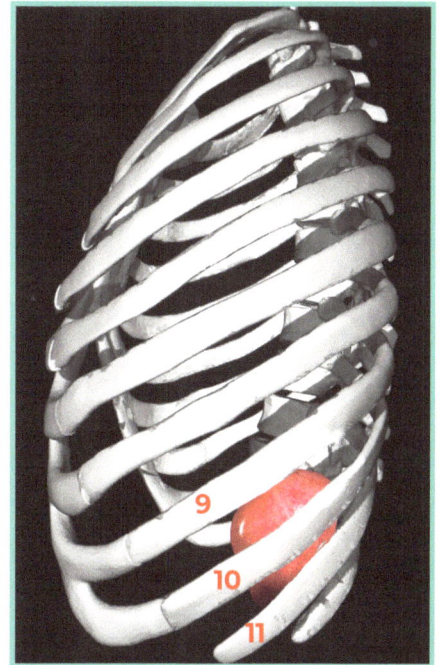

97 Parts of the spleen

> ## Red pulp filters red blood cells.
> ## White pulp stores/activates white blood cells.

The spleen is composed of two main types of tissue: **red pulp** and **white pulp**.

- **Red pulp** filters the blood of worn-out/damaged red blood cells, antigens, and microorganisms.
- **White pulp** carries out various immune functions, like storing and activating B and T cells.

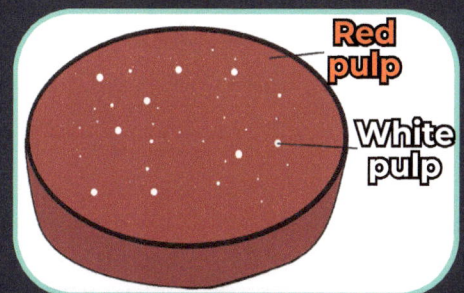

By simply knowing these 2 general functions (*filtration* and *immune functions*), a great deal of spleen pathology can be easily understood:

(!) **Splenomegaly:** Since the spleen filters RBCs and stores WBCs, various problems involving RBCs and WBCs can cause the spleen to get enlarged - called **splenomegaly**. This includes diseases with **abnormal RBC shapes** like thalassemias and early sickle cell disease (the abnormal RBCs clog up the spleen), mononucleosis (*"mono"*), and hematologic cancers like leukemias and lymphomas. Contact sports should be avoided with splenomegaly because of the risk of **splenic rupture**!

(!) **Splenectomy:** Sometimes the spleen has to be removed to treat a splenic disease - called a **splenectomy**. In **sickle cell disease** though, repeated infarctions of the spleen can cause it to shrink and die off *on its own* - called **autosplenectomy**. Patients can live without a spleen but they will be vulnerable to **encapsulated bacteria**.

NOTES

CHAPTER 12

Neurology

98 Ganglion

Ganglion = gang of neurons

A ganglion is a group of **neuron cell bodies** in the **peripheral nervous system**. They serve as **relay points** between different neurological structures in the body, like the central (CNS) and peripheral nervous systems (PNS). They can be grouped into 2 categories:

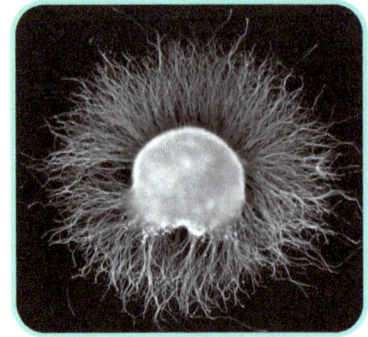
Real image of a dorsal root gaglion.

1) Autonomic ganglia

Contain the cell bodies of **autonomic nerves**.
The nerve fibers from the *CNS* to the *ganglia* are called ***pre*-ganglionic fibers,** while those between the *ganglia* and the *target organ* are called ***post*-ganglionic fibers**.

a) Sympathetic: All sympathetic nerve fibers arise from **T1-L2**. They then synapse onto one of two ganglia:

i) Paravertebral ganglia (**sympathetic chain**): Pearl necklace-like chain **right beside** spinal cord. All sympathetic fibers EXCEPT those going to abdominal or pelvic organs synpase on this chain.

ii) Prevertebral ganglia: Sympathetic fibers going to **all abdominal and pelvic organs** pass through the sympathetic chain *WITHOUT* synapsing, and rather synapse in one of 3 **prevertebral ganglia**. Theses ganglia correspond to the 3 main branches of the abdominal aorta (and are located right by them): the **celiac**, **superior mesenteric**, and **inferior mesenteric ganglia**.

b) Parasympathetic: All parasympathetic nerve fibers arise from **CNs 3, 7, 9, 10 (cranial nerves)** or **S2-4 (pelvic splanchnic nerves).**

(!) Remember that sympathetic ganglia lie **far away** from their target organs, while parasympathetic ganglia lie **close** to them by simply **thinking of the sympathetic chain**, which lies right next to the spinal cord.

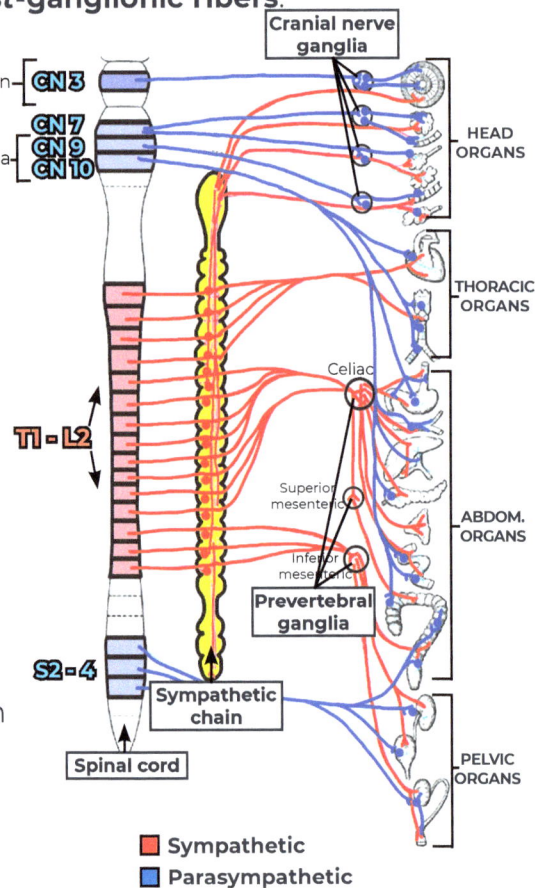

Midbrain — CN 3
Medulla — CN 7 / CN 9 / CN 10
Cranial nerve ganglia
HEAD ORGANS
THORACIC ORGANS
Celiac
T1 - L2
Superior mesenteric
ABDOM. ORGANS
Inferior mesenteric
Prevertebral ganglia
S2-4
Sympathetic chain
Spinal cord
PELVIC ORGANS
■ Sympathetic
■ Parasympathetic

2) Sensory ganglia

Contain the cell bodies of **sensory nerves**. There are 2 main groups of sensory ganglia:

a) Dorsal root ganglia: The majority of the body's sensory nerves have their cell bodies in dorsal root ganglia, which as their name suggests is found in the posterior (dorsal) root right before it enters the spinal cord.

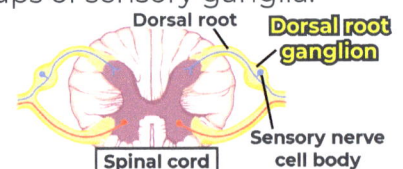
Dorsal root
Dorsal root ganglion
Sensory nerve cell body
Spinal cord

b) Cranial nerve ganglia: Cranial nerve ganglia are essentially the same as the dorsal root ganglia except they involve select *cranial nerves* instead of spinal nerves. Although cranial nerves have their roots inside the skull, their ganglia are actually outside the skull.

99 Grey & white matter

> **Think of the iconic greyish-brown colour of the brain**

Brain

Spinal cord

Remember that...

- **Brain:** grey matter on **OUTSIDE**, white matter on **inside**
- **Spinal cord:** grey matter on **INSIDE**, white matter on **outside**

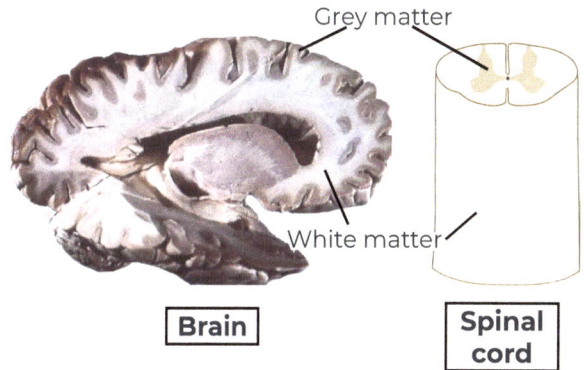

...by simply thinking about that iconic greyish-brown colour of the brain's exterior (which tells you its grey matter is on the *outside*), and then remembering that it is the opposite in the spinal cord (grey matter on *inside*).

The colour difference between grey and white matter is because of the whiteness of **myelin**. Myelin is a material wrapped around axons to speed the transmission of impulses through them. White matter is **mostly axons**, while grey matter is **mostly cell bodies**.

100 Gyrus vs. suclus

> **Alphabetical order, or think "sulk" (feeling down)**

Gyrus

Sulcus

Central sulcus

Parietal lobe

Frontal lobe

Temporal lobe

Occipital lobe

Lateral sulcus

The iconic folded surface of the brain is formed by:

- **Gyri:** the **elevations**
- **Sulci:** the **depressions**

It's easy to forget which is which, so either remember that they follow **alphabetic order** (**G** lies above **S**), or think of the word **"sulk"** (feeling **down**) whenever you read **sulc**us.

Function: Gyri and sulci increase the **surface area** of the brain.

Major sulci: 1. Central sulcus, 2. Lateral sulcus

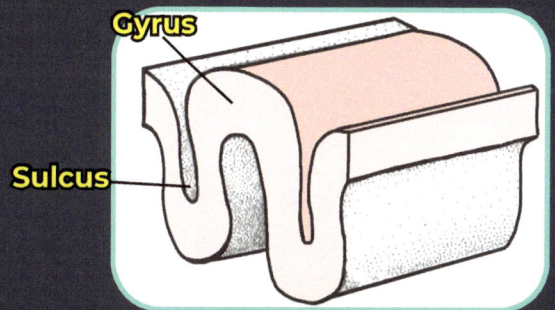

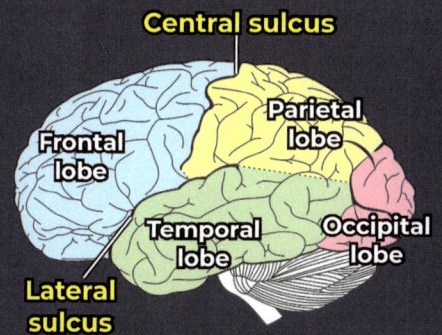

(!) **Lissencephaly**: Meaning **"smooth brain"**, lissencephaly is a set of disorders where the surface of the brain appears smooth because of *absent or abnormally broad gyri*. This is caused by abnormal migration of neurons during gestation. Children with lissencephaly usually have significant developmental delays.

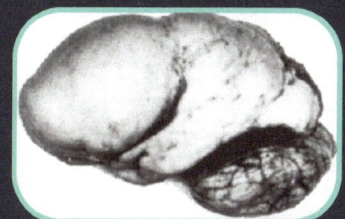

Lissencephaly

101 Cranial nerves

CN 1: Olfactory nerve

> **Stick one finger in your nose (like you're picking it)**

Function: smell (olfaction)

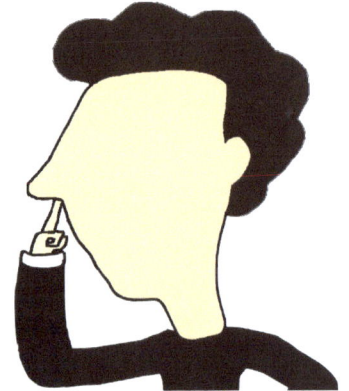

CN 2: Optic nerve

> **Make the "I'm watching you" sign with two fingers**

Function: sight

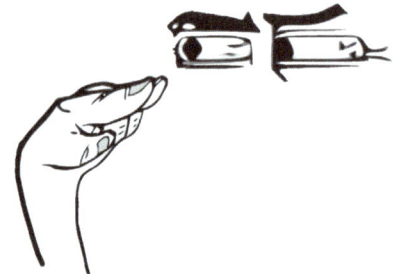

CN 3: Oculomotor nerve

> **Make the "OK" sign with 3 fingers over both eyes to keep your eyelids open (eyelid opening), look around through the holes (MOST eye movement muscles), and squeeze your eyeball (pupillary constriction, accommodation)**

Functions: 1. Eye movement (all ocular muscles except the superior oblique and lateral rectus), 2. eyelid opening, 3. pupillary constriction, 4. accommodation

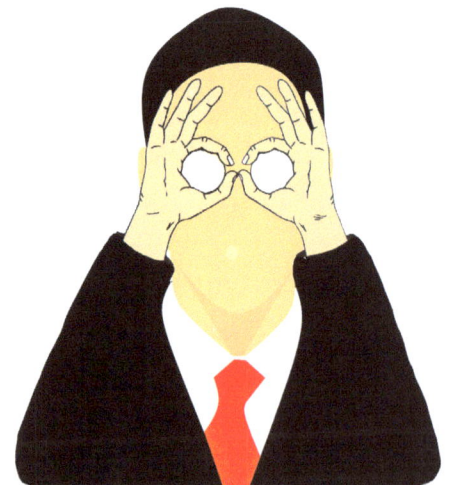

CN 4: Trochlear nerve

"CN **4**: eyes to the **floor**"

Function: eye depression and **intorsion** (via **superior oblique muscle**)

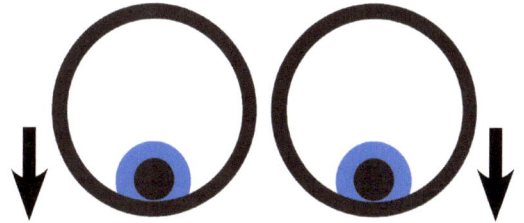

CN 6: Abducens nerve

"CN **6** makes your eyes do the **splits**"

Function: eye abduction (via **lateral rectus muscle**)

Additionally, think of the name '**abducens**' - it literally tells you it **abducts**.

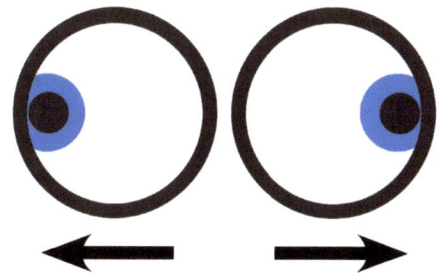

CN 5: Trigeminal nerve

Wipe your **face** and **eat** with your hand (each done with **5** fingers)

Function: 1. Facial sensation (ophthalmic, maxillary, mandibular divisions), **2. Mastication, 3.** Anterior 2/3 of tongue sensation

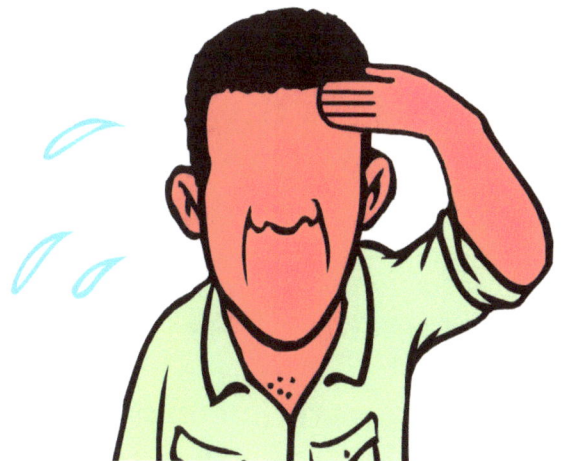

(!) **Trigeminal neuralgia:** Trigeminal neuralgia (*tic douloureux*) is a chronic condition that affects the trigeminal nerve and causes jolts of excruciating facial pain along its path. Even mild stimulation of the face - like brushing one's teeth - can trigger **electric shock-like pain** that lasts a few seconds to a few minutes. It is said to be one of the most painful disorders known in medicine!

CN 7: Facial nerve

Picture someone terrified and crying in fear of the 7 deadly sins (facial expression muscles, lacrimation, salivation). They're closing their eyes in fear (eyelid closing) and plugging their ears (auditory volume modulation).

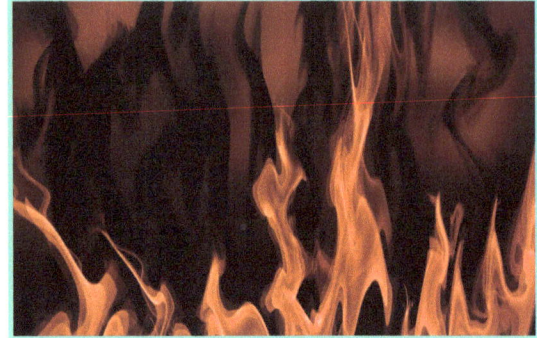

Functions: 1. Facial expression muscles, 2. lacrimation, 3. salivation, 4. eyelid closing, 5. auditory volume modulation (via stapedius muscle), 6. taste from anterior 2/3 of tongue

CN 8: Vestibulocochlear nerve

Make the "I can't hear you" sign with 4 fingers from each hand (4 + 4 = 8)

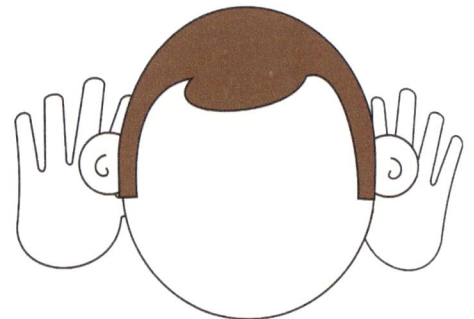

Function: 1. Hearing, 2. Balance

If you can remember CN 8 facilitating hearing, it's easy to remember that it helps with balance as well, as the ear's role in balance is fairly widely known.

(!) **Vertigo:** Conditions that irritate or injure the vestibulocochlear nerve can cause **vertigo** - the sensation that you or the environment around you is **spinning**. Vertigo can be caused by things that affect other parts of the vestibular system too though, like the semilunar canals, vestibule, or even brain and brainstem.

CN 9: Glossopharyngeal nerve

> **Picture a fish hook (looks like a 9) getting stuck in a person's throat**

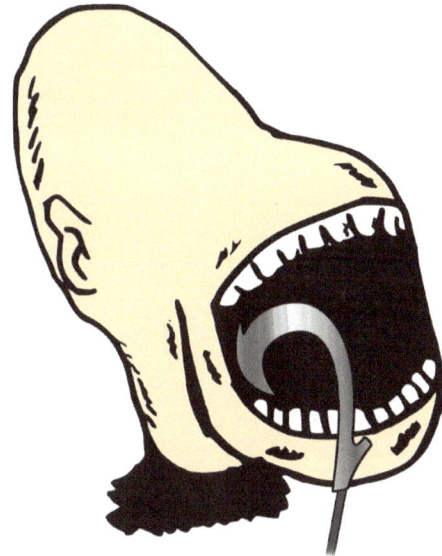

Function: 1. **Swallowing**, 2. **elevation of pharynx/larynx** (stylopharyngeus muscle), 3. **taste and sensation in posterior 1/3 of tongue**, 4. **monitoring carotid body and baro-/chemoreceptors**, 5. **salivation** (parotid gland)

As its name implies, the **glosso-pharyngeal** nerve is all about the **throat** (the *pharynx*) and the (back of the) **tongue** (the *glossus*). Simply think of all the functions that relate to these areas.

CN 10: Vagus nerve

> **"Relaxing vacation in Vegas"**

Function: 1. **Parasympathetics** (*"relaxing"*) to thoracic and abdominal organs, 2. swallowing, 3. soft palate elevation, 4. cough reflex, 5. talking, 6. taste from supraglottic region, 7. monitoring aortic arch baro- /chemoreceptors, 8. keeping u**V**ula midline

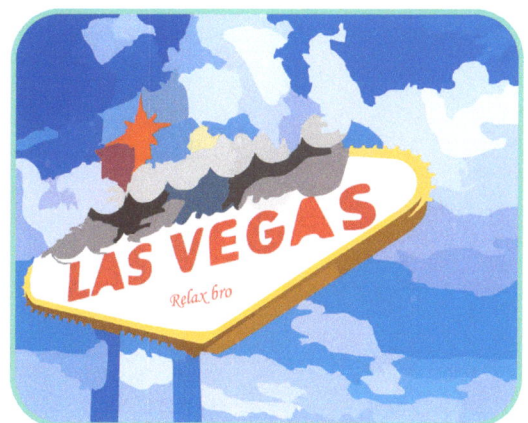

Note: if the vagus nerve is injured, the uvula deviates **AWAY** from the side of the lesion (towards the intact side). Picture the uvula being held in the midline by two strings - one on each side. If the left string is cut (i.e. lesion of left vagus nerve), the right string will pull on the uvula unopposed, causing right uvular deviation.

Vasovagal syncope: Vaso*vagal* syncope is the **most common cause of fainting**. It occurs when a trigger, like emotional stress or the sight of blood, causes **overstimulation of the *vagus* nerve**. This temporarily causes massive parasympathetic stimulation, which decreases blood pressure and slows the heart rate, leading to fainting.

95

CN 11: Accessory nerve

> The trapezius and sternocleidomastoid muscles look like the number 11

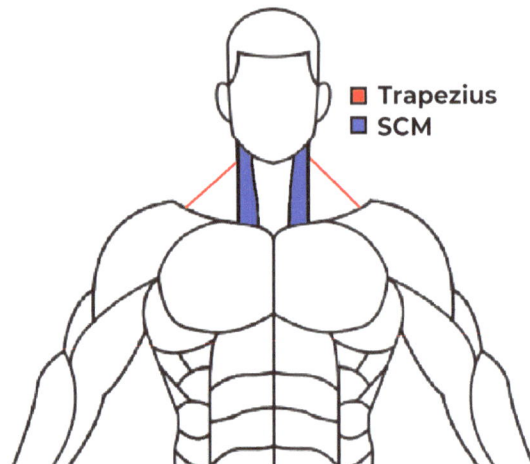

■ Trapezius
■ SCM

Function: 1. Trapezius (shrugging) and **sternocleidomastoid** (head rotation) innervation

CN 12: Hypoglossal nerve

> The last cranial nerve is for language

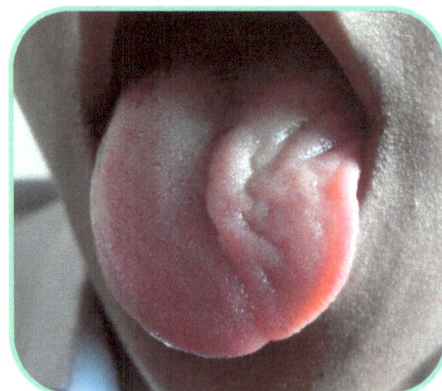

Left hypoglossal nerve lesion.

Function: 1. Tongue movement

Note: if the hypoglossal nerve is injured, the tongue deviates ***TOWARDS*** the side of the lesion (vs. the uvula deviating *AWAY* from the lesion in vagus nerve lesions). Picture the tongue being held out by two muscles like pillars. If you take away one pillar, the tongue caves in towards that side (see image above).

Cranial Nerve Exam Summary

CN 1 (olfactory nerve) is the only cranial nerve not routinely examined in a neurological exam (you don't need to carry around an orange peel or anything) - you can simply ask the patient if they've noticed changes in smell. A very <u>basic</u> examination of CNs 2-12 is as follows:

- **CN 2:** Visual acuity test with Snellen chart
- **CNs 3, 4, and 6:** Assess eye movements (make an 'H' with finger and ask patient to follow)
- **CN 5:** Assess facial sensation with light touch or pin prick (forehead, cheek, and lower jaw)
- **CN 7:** Various facial expressions (raise eyebrows, smile, puff out cheeks, etc.)
- **CN 8:** Whisper a number into each ear, or rub your fingers beside their ear
- **CN 9 and 10:** Ask patient to say 'ah' (soft palate elevating symmetrically = CN 9; uvula midline = CN 10)
- **CN 11:** Shrug shoulders; turn head to the side against resistance
- **CN 12:** Protrude tongue (checking for asymmetry or wasting)

102 Motor vs. sensory cranial nerves

Some Say Marry Money But My Brother Says Big Brains Matter Most

S = Sensory
M = Motor
B = Both (sensory and motor)

CN 1: Sensory
CN 2: Sensory
CN 3: Motor
CN 4: Motor
CN 5: Both
CN 6: Motor

CN 7: Both
CN 8: Sensory
CN 9: Both
CN 10: Both
CN 11: Motor
CN 12: Motor

103 Facial nerve lesions

Upper motor lesions: upper head is spared

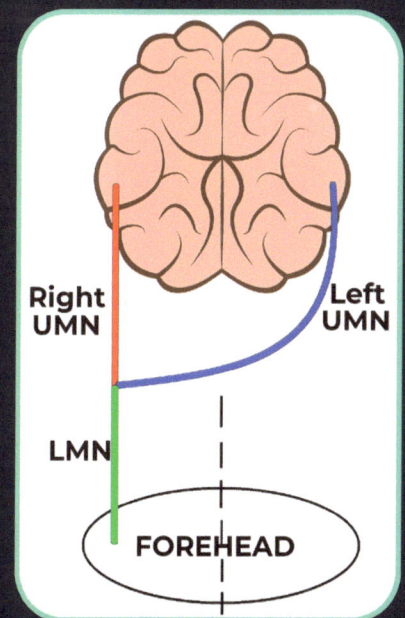

In an **upper motor neuron (UMN)** lesion (e.g. motor cortex), the forehead is spared because it is innervated by **BILATERAL** UMNs. In other words, each side of your forehead is innervated by both the left and right facial nerves, meaning even when there's a lesion (e.g. a stroke) affecting one side of the brain, the other side is still innervating the forehead.

In contrast, a **lower motor neuron (LMN)** lesion (e.g. the facial nerve once it emerges from the brainstem) will cause paralysis of the entire face, including the forehead, because it injures the nerve _after_ the bilateral UMNs have joined together (at which point it's called the facial nerve - a LMN).

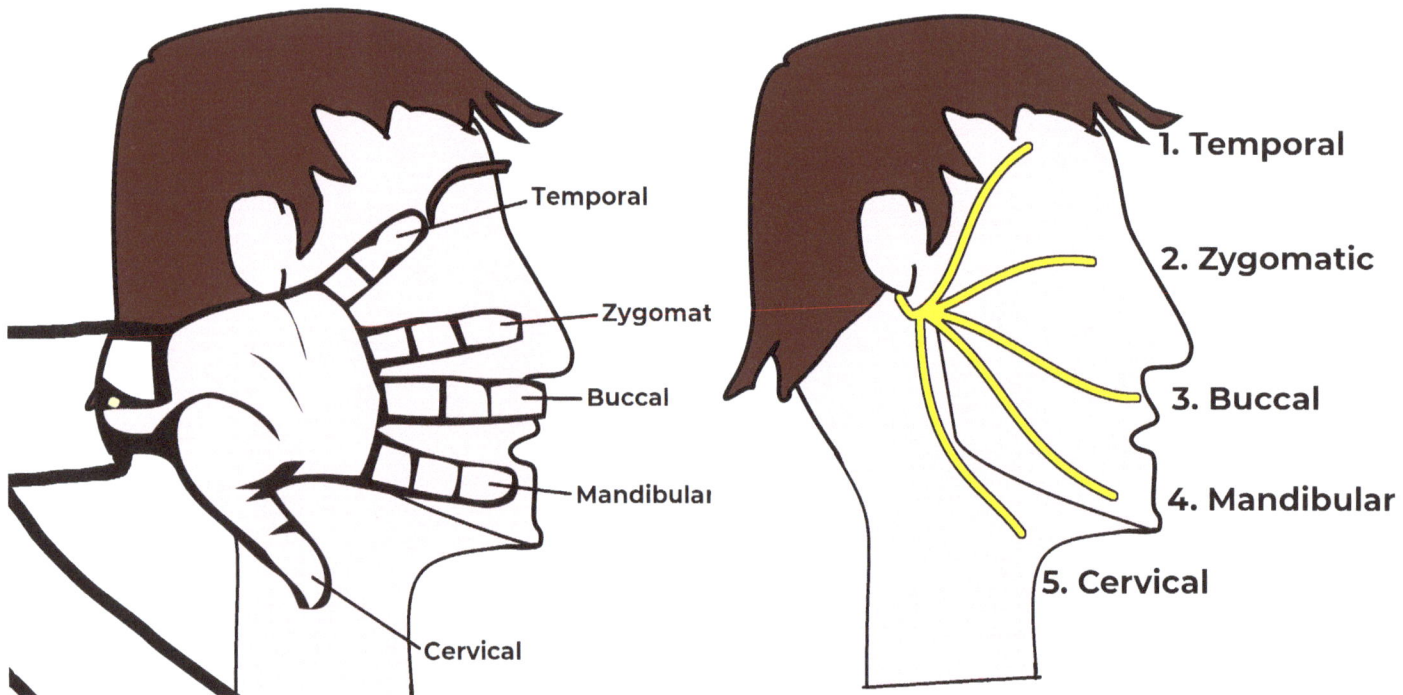

Temporal

Zygomat

Buccal

Mandibular

Cervical

1. Temporal

2. Zygomatic

3. Buccal

4. Mandibular

5. Cervical

104 **Facial nerve - motor branches**

Reverse facepalm

As seen in the image above, press your hand backwards against your face like an idiot and your fingers will naturally align with the 5 branches of the facial nerve.

To remember the name of each branch, simply think of the area in which the nerve lies.

- **Temporal**: along your **temple**
- **Zygomatic**: Right over your **zygomatic bone** (see *Bones of the Face* mnemonic)
- **Buccal**: 'buccal' means **mouth**
- **Mandibular**: along your **mandible**
- **Cervical**: by your **cervical spine** (i.e. neck)

wut am i doing lol

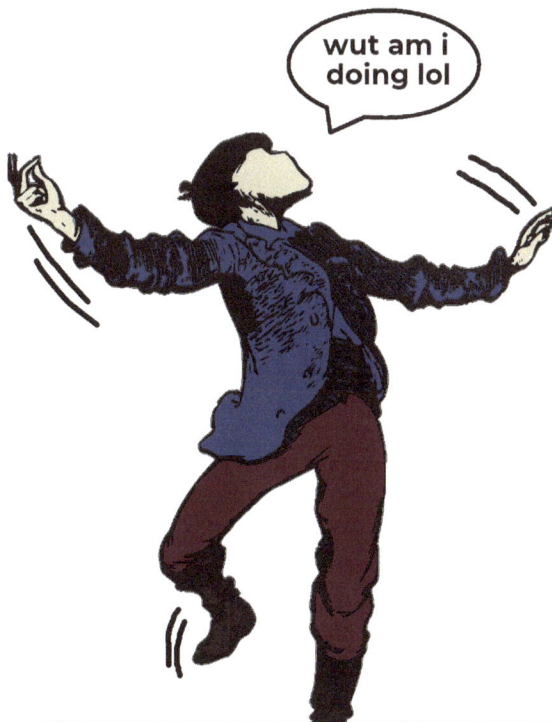

Nucleus ambiguus

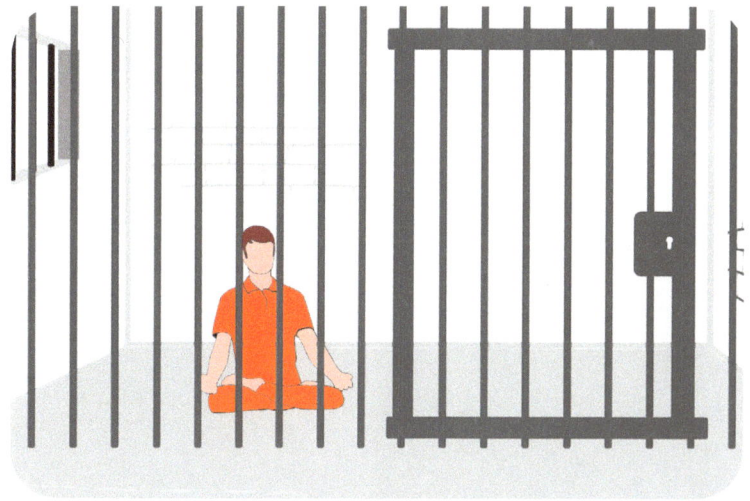

Nucleus solitarius

105 Vagal nuclei

The vagal nuclei are nuclei in the **medulla** that serve as the "roots" of the **vagus nerve (CN 10)**. Axons from these nuclei all converge to form the vagus nerve that we all know and love. There are **3 main vagal nuclei**:

1. **Nucleus ambiguus: motor innervation**
   - Picture making **ambiguous motor** movements
2. **Nucleus solitarius: sensory innervation**
   - Picture the heightened **senses** you experience when in **solitary** confinement
3. **Dorsal motor nucleus: autonomic (parasympathetic)**
   - Motor and sensory are already taken, so it must be autonomic

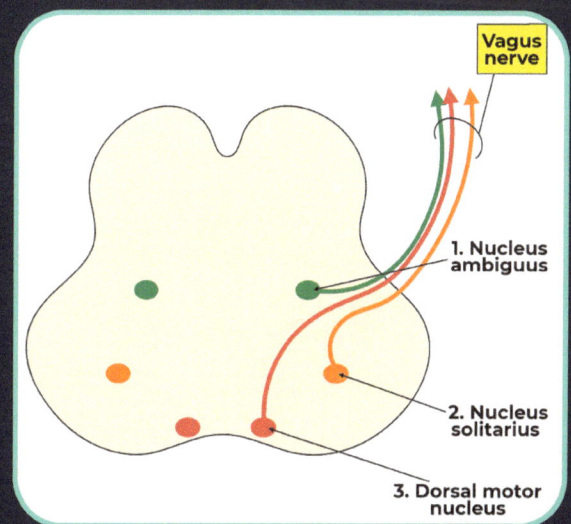

Alternatively, you can use this mnemonic:

Vagus nerve

1. Nucleus ambiguus

2. Nucleus solitarius

3. Dorsal motor nucleus

**Nucleus Solitarius: Sensory
Nucleus aMbiguus: Motor**

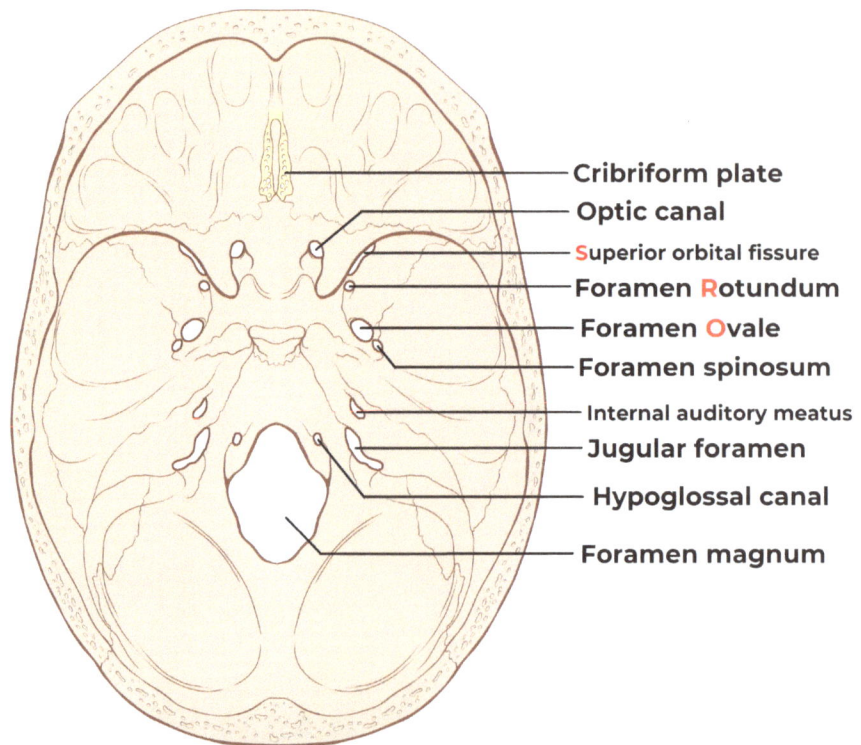

- Cribriform plate
- Optic canal
- **S**uperior orbital fissure
- Foramen **R**otundum
- Foramen **O**vale
- Foramen spinosum
- Internal auditory meatus
- Jugular foramen
- Hypoglossal canal
- Foramen magnum

106 Cranial foramina & contents

1. **Cribriform plate: CN 1 (olfactory nerve)**
   - Imagine someone's **smelly crib**
2. **Optic canal: CN 2 (optic nerve), ophthalmic artery**
   - It probably won't come as a shock that the **optic** canal contains perhaps the two most important structures for vision - the **optic** nerve and the **ophthalmic** artery
3. **Superior orbital fissure: CNs 3, 4, 6, and V1 (from CN 5)**
   - Superior **orbital** fissure contains all 3 nerves that move your eyeball around in your **orbit**
   - This is a **FISSURE** – not just a foramen like the rest. Hence it understandably is large and contains many structures
4. **Locations of the 3 branches of CN V:** **SRO**
   - **S**uperior orbital fissure: V1
   - Foramen **R**otundum: V2
   - Foramen **O**vale: V3
5. **Internal auditory meatus: CN 7, CN 8**
   - As its name implies, the internal auditory meatus contains the two nerves that deal with **hearing** (CN 8 receives auditory information, CN 7 innervates the stapedius muscle in the ear which contracts to modulate volume).
6. **Jugular foramen: Jugular vein + CN 9, 10, and 11**
   - *"9, 10, 11 – jugular foramen"*
   - The jugular foramen looks long and floppy/tortuous, just like the jugular vein
7. **Hypoglossal canal: Hypoglossal nerve (CN 12)**
8. **Foramen magnum: Brainstem + vertebral arteries**
   - '**Magnum**' means *big/great* – so it's only befitting that it houses the most massive structure of any foramen: the brainstem
   - It makes sense that traveling within the **VERTBERAL column** alongside the brainstem/spinal cord are the **VERTEBRAL** arteries to supply them with blood.

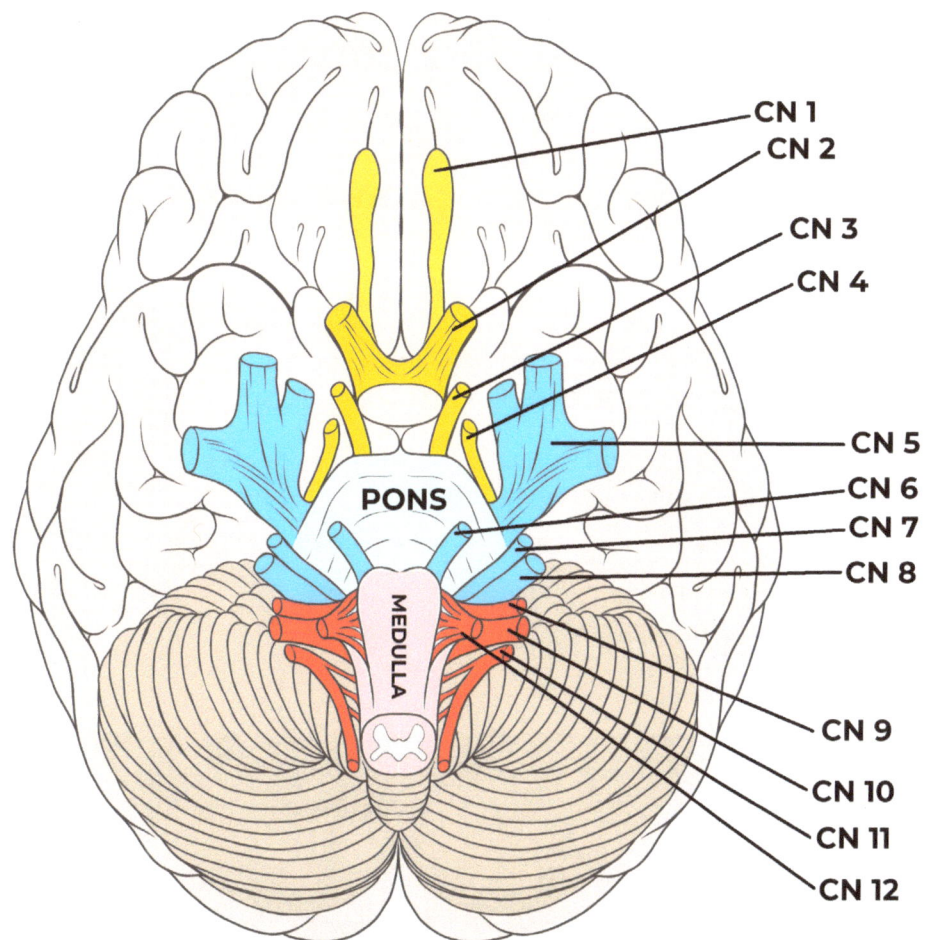

CN 1
CN 2
CN 3
CN 4
CN 5
CN 6
CN 7
CN 8
CN 9
CN 10
CN 11
CN 12
PONS
MEDULLA

107 Emergence of cranial nerves

4 CNs are above the pons (1, 2, 3, 4)
4 CNs are in the pons (5, 6, 7, 8)
4 CNs are in the medulla (9, 10, 11, 12)
4 CN nuclei are medial (3, 4, 6, 12)
  • "Factors of 12, except 1 and 2"

CN 1 (olfactory nerve) and **CN 2 (optic nerve)** are the only two nerves that emerge from the **cerebrum** - the rest emerge from the **brainstem** (CN 3 and 4 emerge from the midbrain).

By knowing the locations of cranial nerves, you can get an idea of where in the brain or brainstem a stroke might have occured just by performing a cranial nerve exam!

108 Motor vs. sensory cortex

> The **motor** of a car is at its **anterior** end

Similarly:

- **Motor** cortex: **anterior** to central sulcus
- **Sensory cortex: posterior** to central sulcus

Remember that it's the **central sulcus** that divides the two because it's literally called the **central** sulcus (i.e. at the center of the two).

Bonus: The **pre-motor cortex**, as its name implies, comes **before** (i.e. just anterior to) the motor cortex.

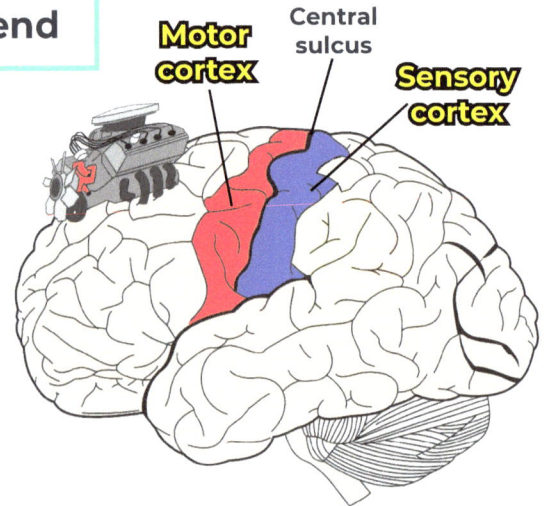

109 Anterior vs. posterior horn of spinal cord

> Again...the **motor** of a car is at its **anterior** end

There are 3 grey matter "horns" in the spinal cord: **anterior** (ventral), **posterior** (dorsal), and **lateral**. These horns are simply areas where *cell bodies* of specific neurons lie.

The anterior and posterior horns of the spinal cord share the *same pattern as the motor and sensory cortices of the brain*: motor function lies anterior and sensory lies posterior. Therefore:

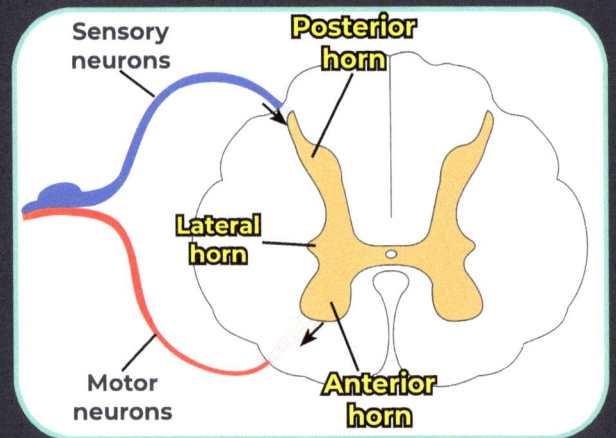

- **Anterior** horn: **motor** neurons
- **Posterior** horn: sensory neurons

- Lateral horn: symathetic neurons (only exists at T1-L2)

(!) **Anterior horn destruction: Amyotrophic lateral sclerosis (ALS)** and **poliomyelitis (*"polio"*)** destroy the anterior horn, resulting in paralysis.

110 Conus medullaris vs. cauda equina vs. filum terminale

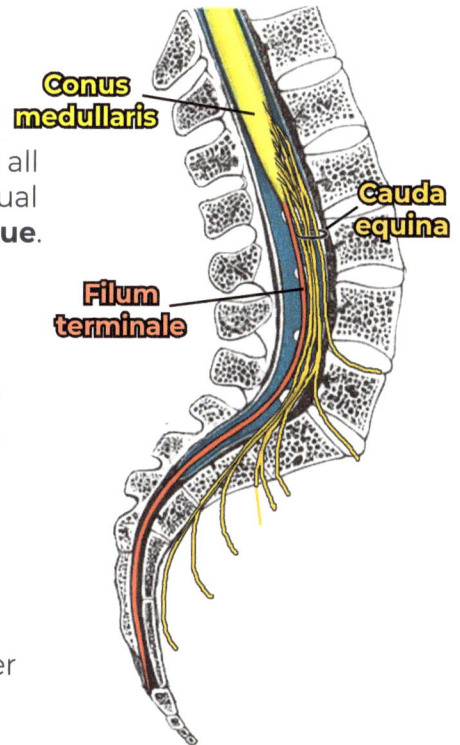

Conus medullaris

Cauda equina

Filum terminale

In the name

The conus medullaris, cauda equina, and filum terminale are all structures near the bottom end of the spinal cord. One is actual **spinal cord**, one is **peripheral nerves**, and one is **fibrous tissue**.

Nervous tissue

- **Conus medullaris:** simply the bottom (**cone**) end of the **spinal cord**. Since this is *actual spinal cord*, it has **upper motor neurons (UMN)**. It ends around the level of **L1-L2**.
- **Cauda equina** (*"horse's tail"*): **peripheral nerves** (**lower motor neurons [LMN]**) extending out from the conus medullaris like a horse's tail. Nerves L2 and onward.

NOT nervous tissue

- **Filum terminale** (*"terminal thread"*): **fibrous tissue** after the **termination** of the spinal cord

! **Lumbar puncture:** Lumbar punctures are performed at the level of **L3-L4** to avoid injuring the spinal cord because it ends at L1-L2. The needle doesn't injure the cauda equina - it simply pushes them aside!

! **Cauda equina syndrome vs. conus medullaris syndrome:** Compression (e.g. tumor) can injure the cauda equina or conus medullaris, resulting in their respective syndromes. Since the conus medullaris is an UMN, conus medullaris syndrome causes **UMN symptoms** (symmetric, hyperreflexia, fasciculations) while cauda equina syndrome causes **LMN symptoms** (asymmetric, areflexia, flaccid paralysis).

111 Thalamic nuclei

A) Lateral vs. medial geniculate nuclei

- **Lateral:** senses **Light** (i.e. vision)
- **Medial:** senses **Music** (i.e. hearing)

B) Ventral postero-lateral (VPL) vs. ventral postero-medial (VPM) nuclei

- **VPL:** senses **Vibration, Pain, Pressure, Proprioception, Light touch, temperature**
- **VPM:** senses **taste**, face sensation ("VP**M**mmmmm....")

*These are only select important nuclei. The thalamus has a large number of nuclei, but in most cases it is not necessary to memorize them all.

103

112 Meninges

Dura mater: durable outermost layer

Arachnoid mater: middle layer with web-like connections that absorb CSF
- *'Arachnoid'* (like *arachnid*) literally refers to its **spider web**-like connections and protrusions, which function to absorb cerebrospinal fluid.

Pia mater: thin, delicate inner layer that adheres to the brain and spinal cord like the delicate crust of a **pie**

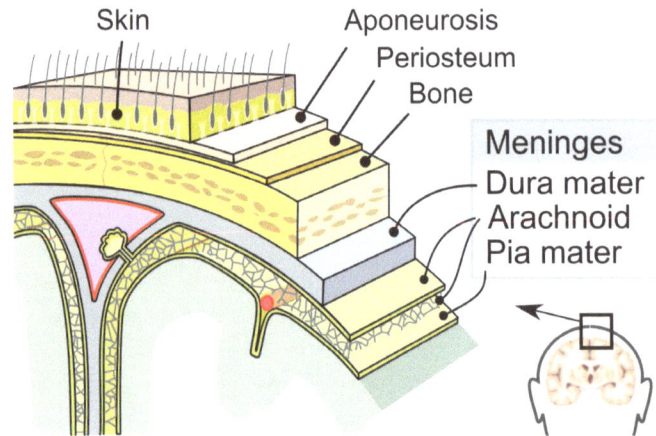

Skin — Aponeurosis — Periosteum — Bone

Meninges
Dura mater
Arachnoid
Pia mater

*

! **Meningitis** is an inflammation of the meninges, usually from infection by bacteria or viruses. Viral meningitis is less severe and usually does not require specific treatment, but bacterial meningitis is life-threatening!

113 Important dermatome landmarks

- **T4: at the nipple ("T4 at the teat pore")**
- **T10: at the umbilicus ("T10 at the belly butTEN")**
- **L1: at the inguinal ligament (L1 = IL [Inguinal Ligament])**
- **L4: includes the kneecaps ("crawling on ALL 4's [L4]")**

Referred pain: *Referred pain* is pain perceived at a location other than the site of the painful stimulus. This happens when visceral (internal organ) and somatic pain fibers converge on the same ascending tract (spinothalamic tract) in the spinal cord. When the internal organ feels pain, the brain thus interprets that signal as coming from the body surface. Examples include:

- **Myocardial infarctions** causing left shoulder and jaw pain
- **Acute cholecystitis** causing right shoulder pain
- **Splenic injury** that irritates the diaphragm induces pain in the left shoulder tip (**Kehr's sign**)

Shingles (herpes zoster): *Shingles* is a disease in which the **varicella zoster virus (VZV)** (the chickenpox virus) is reactivated in the body, leading to a severely painful, blistering rash **along a dermatome.** This happens because once the primary infection of VZV is cleared, the virus remains dormant in the **dorsal root ganglia.** When the immune system becomes weakened (e.g. old age), the virus can reactivate and irritate the nerve. Therefore, if you see a painful, *UNILATERAL* rash *along a dermatome* in an elderly or HIV patient, think shingles!

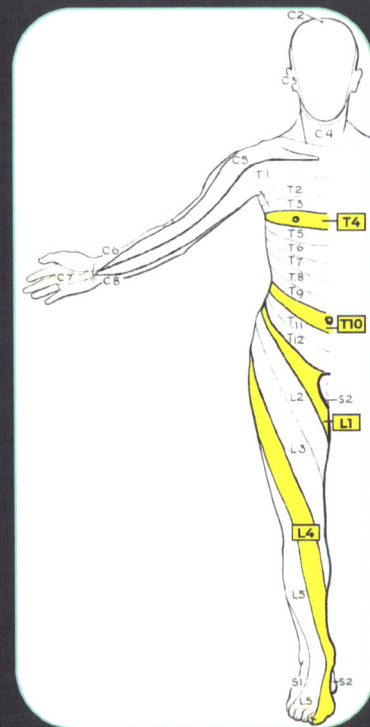

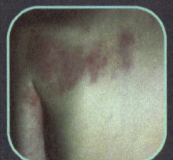

Shingles rash along the C8 dermatome

CERVICAL

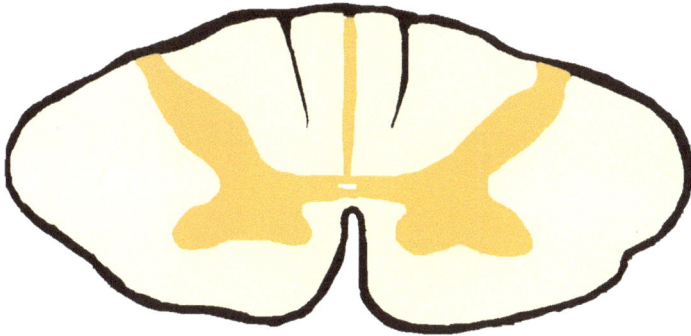

THORACIC

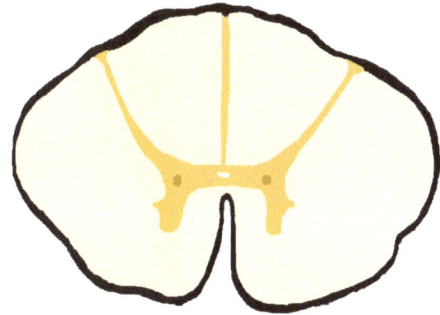

LUMBAR

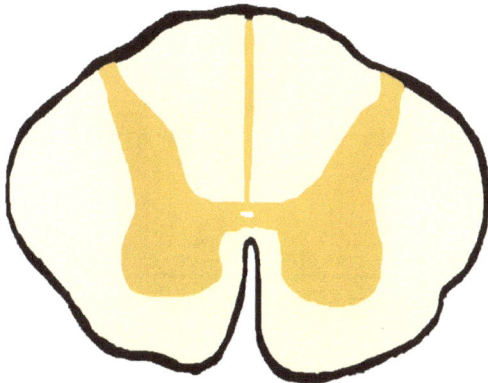

SACRAL

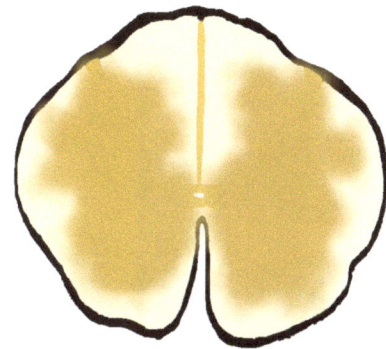

114 **Spinal cord cross sections**

Cervical: Very wide laterally
- Easy to understand and remember why: the cervical spinal cord is the first structure after the brainstem, which is a much wider structure than the spinal cord.
- Additionally, think: "**Curve-ical**"

Thoracic: Very thin grey matter + "tiger eyes"
- **T**horacic grey matter is very thin, just like the letter '**T**' looks thin
- Within the thoracic grey matter are two dots (called the *dorsal nucleus*) that make the thoracic grey matter look like a **t**iger

Lumbar: Much fatter grey matter than the thoracic spinal cord
- Just like your body fat accumulates in your lumbar region and you get a big belly, the lumbar grey matter likewise is much fatter than its thoracic counterpart.

Sacral: "Looks like crap, which should remind you of where you are"

SPINA BIFIDA

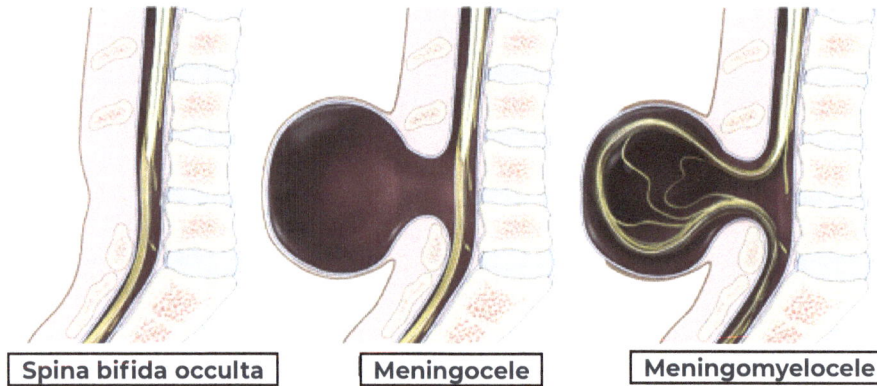

| Spina bifida occulta | Meningocele | Meningomyelocele |

ENCEPHALOCELE

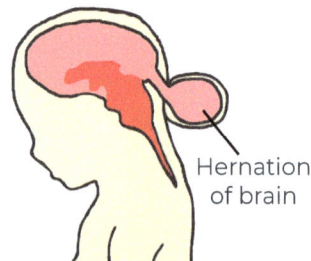

Hernation
of brain

ANENCEPHALY

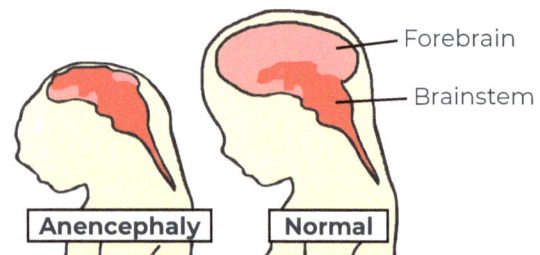

Forebrain

Brainstem

| Anencephaly | Normal |

115 **Neural tube defects**

The names tell you exactly what the disease is

IN THE NAME!

Neural tube defects are a group of birth defects in which the **neural tube** - an opening in the brain and spinal cord that is present in early development - remains open. They are associated with **low folate (vitamin B9)** intake before conception and during pregnancy. They include:

A) Spina bifida

1. **Spina bifida occulta: spine** defect with **NO herniation**
   • ('**occulta**' means *hidden*)
2. **Meningocele:** Spine defect with **herniation** of the **meninges**
   • '**Meningo-**' = meninges; '**-cele**' = herniation
3. **Meningomyelocele:** Spine defect with **herniation** (-**cele**) of **meninges** (**meningo**-) AND **neural tissue** (**myelo**-)

B) Encephalocele

Herniation (-**cele**) of the **brain** (**encephalo-**) through a sac-like protrusion in the skull

C) Anencephaly

Absence (**a-**) of a **forebrain** (-**encephaly**) and part of the skull

116 Holoprosencephaly

"**Whole**-o-prosencephaly"

Holoprosencephaly is a birth defect where the **right and left brain hemispheres fail to separate**.

'**Holo-**' literally means '**whole**', and '**-prosencephaly**' means '**relating to the forebrain (i.e. cerebral hemispheres)**'. This name tells you exactly what the issue is – your cerebral hemispheres remain **WHOLE** rather than separating into left and right hemispheres.

B Holoprosencephaly may be related to mutations in the **sonic hedgehog signaling pathway**. Try vividly picturing the cartoon figure Sonic the Hedgehog slicing the brain in two.

117 Syringomyelia

"**Syringe**-o-myelia"

Syringomyelia is a condition in which a **cystic cavity** (a "**syrinx**") forms within the **central canal** of the spinal cord

The name again tells you exactly what the issue is: '*syringo-*' means *tube* (as in *syringe*) and '*-myelia*' means *neural tissue*.

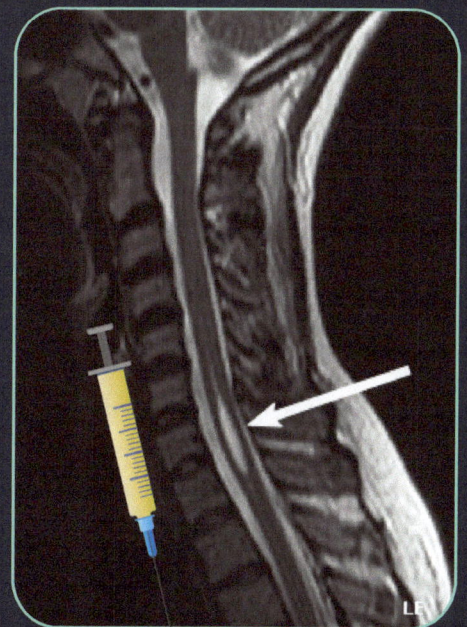

B Syringomyelia causes **bilateral loss of pain and temperature** sensation because it compresses and damages the crossing fibers of the **spinothalamic tract**. Think: "**with syringomyelia you won't be able to feel the pain of a syringe**".

118 Hypothalamus

a) Lateral area: causes hunger. Destruction = anorexia, failure to thrive (infants)
- "If you zap your **lateral** area, you shrink **laterally**"

b) Ventromedial area: causes satiety. Destruction = hyperphagia.
- "If you zap your **ventromedial** area, you grow **ventrally** and **medially**"

c) Anterior hypothalamus: causes cooling, parasympathetic stimulation.
- "**A/C = anterior cooling**"
- Logically makes sense that cooling is done by parasympathetic stimulation (think *"rest and digest"*)

d) Posterior hypothalamus: simply the opposite of the anterior hypothalamus (causes **heating, sympathetic stimulation**)
- Logically makes sense that sympathetic stimulation gets you heated up (think *"fight or flight"*)

e) Suprachiasmatic nucleus: circadian rhythm
- "You need good **sleep** to be **charismatic** (**chiasmatic**)".

119 Superior vs. inferior colliculi

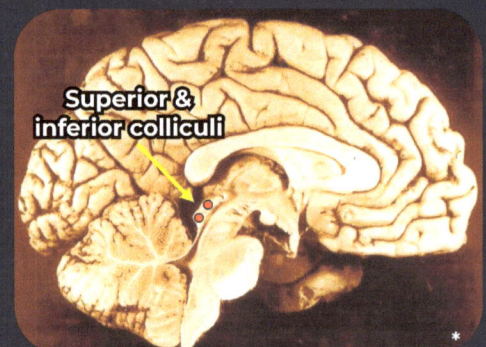

Thalamus

Superior colliculi

Inferior colliculi

Medulla

Posterior view of brainstem

> **Your eyes are located more superiorly than your ears**

- **Superior colliculi: conjugate vertical gaze**
- **Inferior colliculi: auditory**

Just as your **eyes** are situated more **superiorly** than your **ears** (most of it at least), coordination of **eye** movements is done by the **superior colliculus**, while the **inferior colliculus** serves as the center for receiving **auditory signals**. Both are located in the **midbrain**.

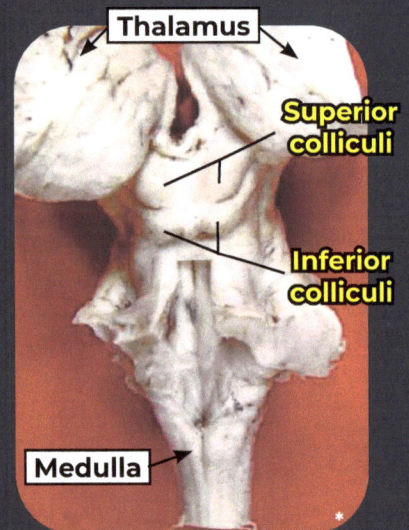

Superior & inferior colliculi

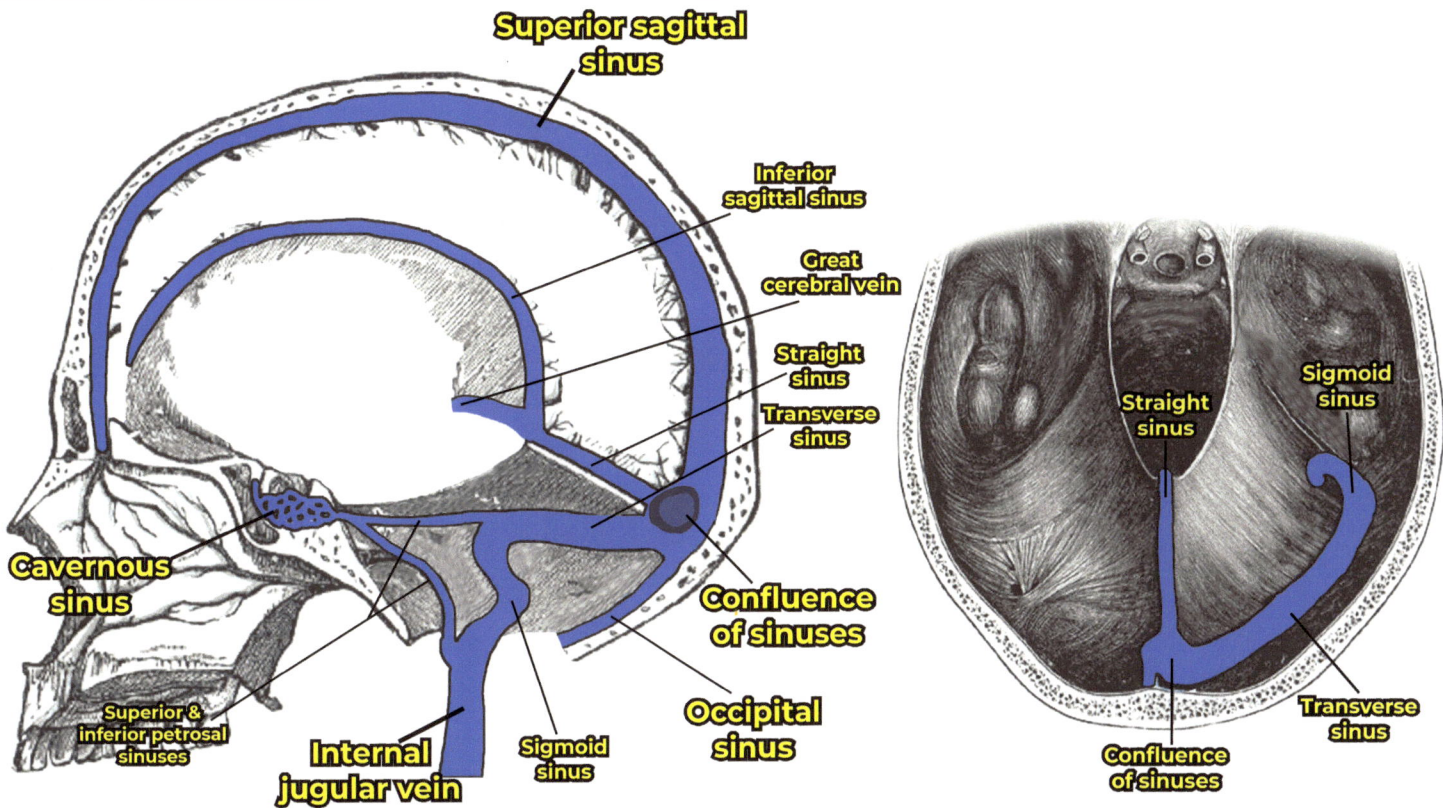

Superior sagittal sinus

Inferior sagittal sinus

Great cerebral vein

Straight sinus

Transverse sinus

Cavernous sinus

Confluence of sinuses

Superior & inferior petrosal sinuses

Internal jugular vein

Sigmoid sinus

Occipital sinus

Straight sinus

Sigmoid sinus

Transverse sinus

Confluence of sinuses

120 Venous drainage of the brain

<u>Overarching idea:</u> The **superior sagittal**, **inferior sagittal**, and **occipital sinuses** and the **great cerebral vein** ultimately end up becoming the **internal jugular vein**. The **transverse** and **sigmoid sinuses** are basically the internal jugular vein <u>*before it leaves the skull*</u>. Then simply remember that the **cavernous sinus** dumps in some blood towards the very end.

1. <u>Superior and inferior sagittal sinuses</u>: As their names imply, these travel along the **sagittal** plane. Obviously the former lies **superiorly** and the latter **inferiorly**.
2. <u>Great cerebral vein</u>: "*Great*" because it penetrates right to the brain's very core.
3. <u>Straight sinus</u>: **Straight** path to the confluence of sinuses
4. <u>Confluence of sinuses</u>: **Con**necting point of the 1) superior sagittal sinus, 2) straight sinus, and 3) occipital sinus.
5. Transverse sinus: Travels out along the **transverse** plane (i.e. laterally).
6. Sigmoid sinus: The winding water slide right before the system exits the skull as the internal jugular vein (via the jugular foramen). '**Sigmoid**' means '**S-shaped**'.
7. Occipital sinus: Originates from **occiput**.
8. Cavernous sinus: Network of many small '**caves**' at the very base of the brain (think: *deep caves!*).
9. Superior and inferior petrosal sinuses: Think '*pumps **petro**lium out of the deep **caves** (cavernous sinus)*'.

(!) **Cavernous sinus thrombosis:** Nearby infection (e.g. in the nose, sinuses, ears, or teeth) can find its way into the cavernous sinus because of interconnecting venous drainage. This can cause thrombosis (blood clot) in the cavernous sinus, which can cause blindness, cranial nerves paralysis, meningitis, and even death!

121 Drawing the circle of Willis

Draw an angry ant

The **circle of Willis** is a system of anastomosing (joining) arteries that lie at the base of the brain. The **internal carotid artery** and the **vertebral artery** are the two arteries that supply blood to the brain, and the circle of Willis is what joins these two systems. It conveniently looks like an angry ant:

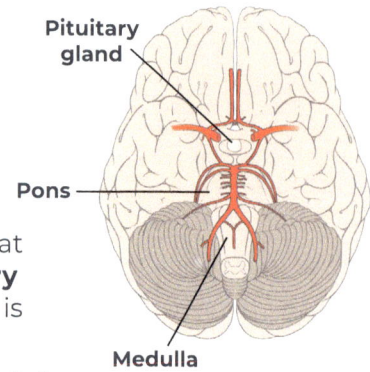

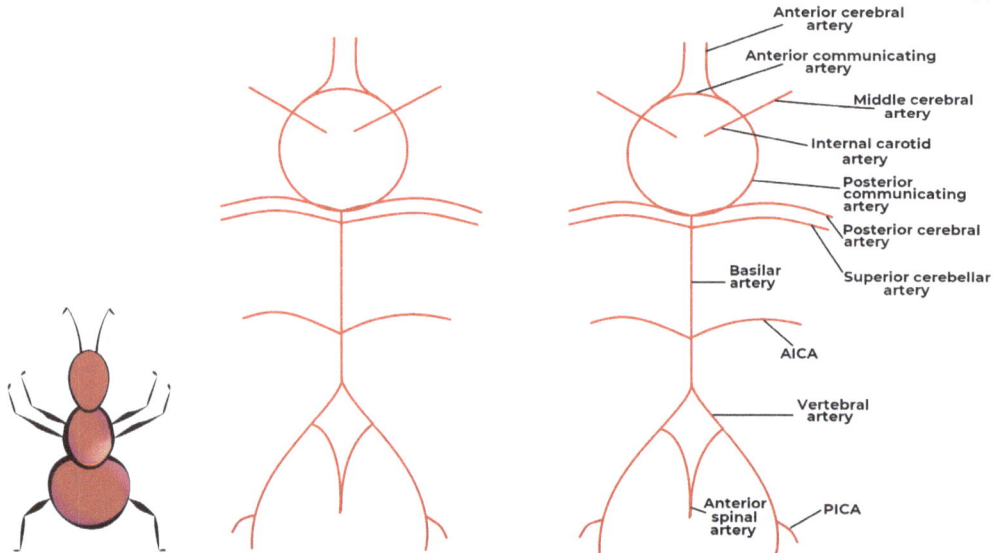

Pituitary gland
Pons
Medulla

Anterior cerebral artery
Anterior communicating artery
Middle cerebral artery
Internal carotid artery
Posterior communicating artery
Posterior cerebral artery
Superior cerebellar artery
Basilar artery
AICA
Vertebral artery
Anterior spinal artery
PICA

122 Cerebellum

- **Medial cerebellum:** coordination of **medial**/midline parts of the body (i.e. trunk, proximal limbs).
- **Lateral cerebellum:** coordination of **lateral** parts of the body (i.e. extremities).

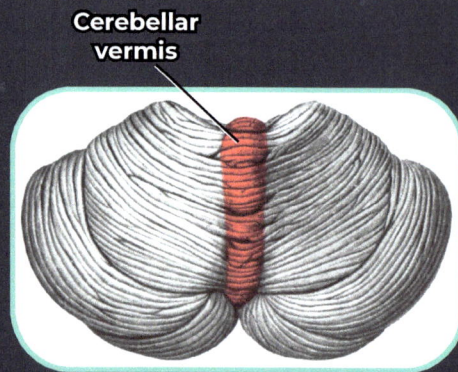

Cerebellar vermis

Cerebellar vermis, a lesion to which causes truncal ataxia

Medial cerebellar lesions (vermal cortex, fastigial nuclei, and flocculonodular lobe) cause truncal ataxia (wide-based gait), head-tilting, and nystagmus (repetitive, involuntary eye movements).

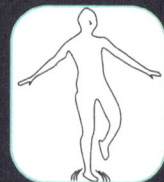

Lateral cerebellar lesions cause problems with extremity coordination (i.e. limb ataxia) and a tendency to fall towards the injured side.

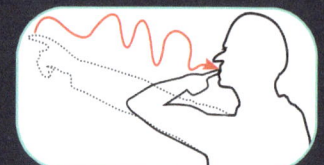

Truncal ataxia due to medial cerebellar lesion.

Abnormal finger-to-nose test showing **limb ataxia** due to lateral cerebellar lesion.

123 Glial cells

Glial cells, or neuroglia, are the supportive cells of the nervous system. The central nervous system (CNS) has 4 types of glial cells, while the peripheral nervous system (PNS) has 2. To remember which belong to which system, simply remember the 2 PNS cells - **Schwann cells** and **satellite cells**. You can do this by thinking of the **"SS (ship prefix) sailing off into the periphery"**. Everything else belongs to the CNS (none start with 'S').

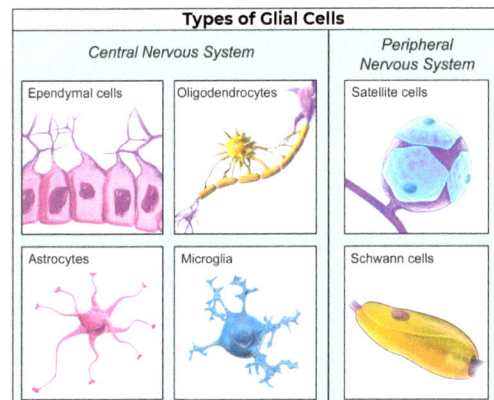

Types of Glial Cells

A) CNS cells

1. Astrocytes: "Astro-" should make you think of the **general fabric** of the universe (**"astronomy"**). Similarly, astrocytes serve **physical/mechanical roles** (physical support, removes excess neurotransmitters, component of blood-brain barrier, repair/reactive gliosis after neural injury).

2. Microglia: the only glial cell with **"micro-"** in its name, hence it's befitting that its role is as a **scavenger** in the CNS – they eat away at dead tissue like **microorganisms**.
  - *BONUS:* **HIV-infected microglia fuse to form multinucleated giant cells** (think: "HIV makes microglia become **MACRO**glia").

3. Oligodendrocytes: think **"oligo my eggo!"**. Oligodendrocytes **wrap myelin around axons** like they're **eggos**. Additionally, the letter **'O'** in 'Oligodendrocyte' should remind you of its **round, spinning function**.
  - *BONUS:* **'Oligo-'** means **'a few'** – so remember that oligodendrocytes can myelinate **MULTIPLE** axons (~30), compared to Schwann cells which only myelinate 1 PNS axon.

4. Ependymal cells: serve as the **epithelial lining of the ventricles.**

B) PNS cells

There are only 2 PNS glial cells, so simply remember that **Schwann cells myelinate axons** (like **oligodendrocytes**) and **satellite cells** are essentially the **astrocytes of the PNS**. No need for mnemonics here.

124 Sensory receptors

1. Meissner corpuscles: sense **fine, light touch**
- "**My Sinner's** corpuscles" (get what I mean by **'fine, light touch'**?)

2. Pacinian corpuscles: sense **pressure** and **vibration**
- Picture **Manny Pacquiao's punches** (you feel their **pressure** and **vibration** as they hit you)

3. Merkel discs: sense **pressure**
- "**Merkel** (German politician) can handle great political **pressure**"

4. Ruffini corpuscles: located at finger tips and joints – sense **pressure** and **slippage of objects** along the surface of skin
- Picture feeling a **Ruffle's** chip slipping out of your fingers.

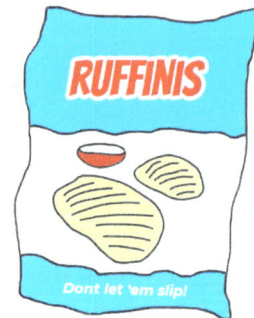

5. Free nerve endings: sense pain and temperature

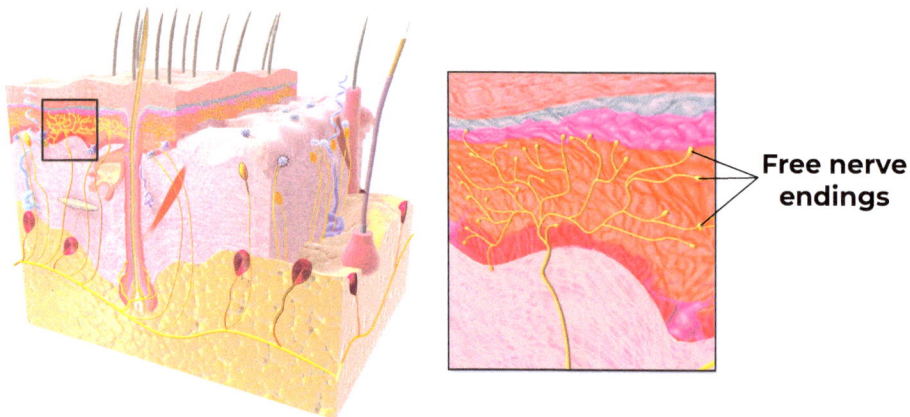

CHAPTER 13

Respiratory

125   Lung lobes

The right lung has <u>3 lobes</u> while the left has <u>2</u> because the heart lies more on the left and takes up the space – hence there is only space for 2 lobes.

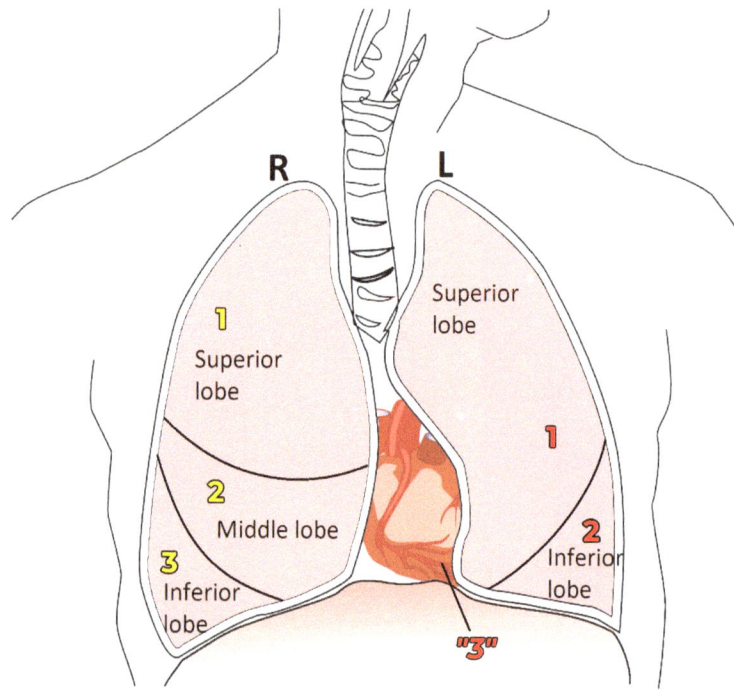

! Knowledge of the lobes of the lung is clinically important for several reasons, like being able to recognize lobar pneumonia (pneumonia localized to one lung lobe) on x-ray.

R   L

1 Superior lobe

Superior lobe

1

2 Middle lobe

2 Inferior lobe

3 Inferior lobe

"3"

REMINDER   Innervation of the diaphragm: **"C3-5 keeps the diaphragm alive!"** (Ch. 5)

126   Lingula

The Lingula Licks the heart

The **lingula** is a projection of the **left lung** at its inferior anteromedial. Its name literally means **"little tongue"**, and it looks just like one too. It slithers right around and in front of the heart.

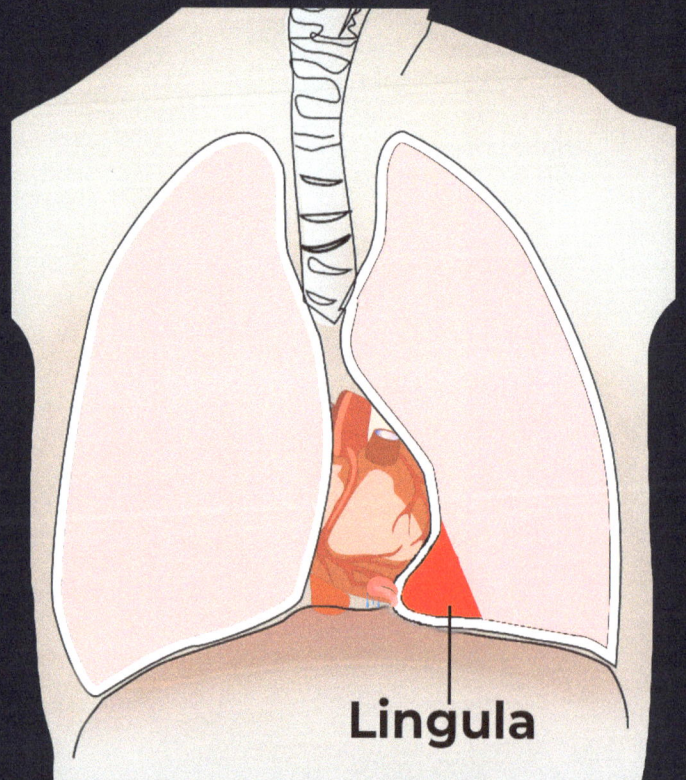

IN THE NAME!

Lingula

127 Lung root/hilum

A) Pulmonary arteries vs. veins

> **The pulmonary arteries lie above the pulmonary veins.**

The **hilum** of the lung is the depression in the medial part of the lung where the pulmonary vessels and bronchus enter.

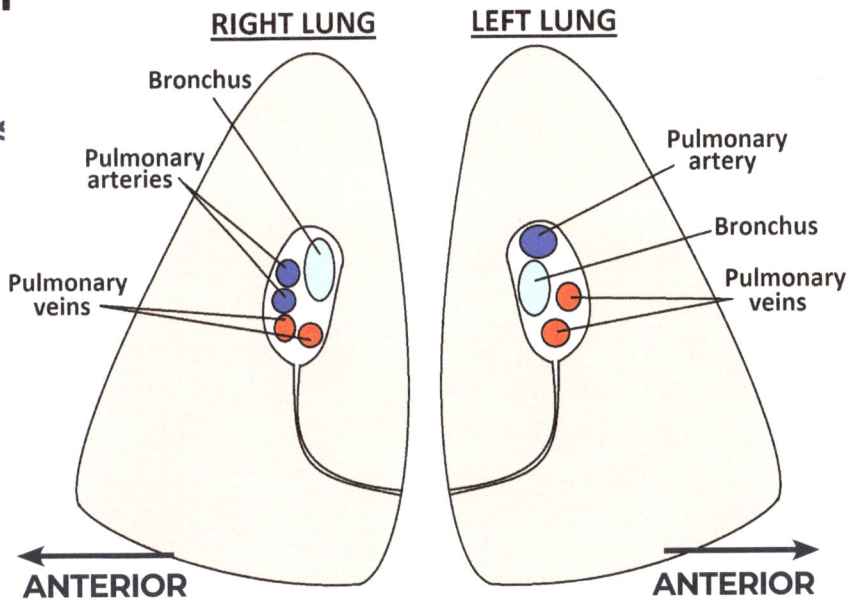

RIGHT LUNG   **LEFT LUNG**

Bronchus

Pulmonary arteries

Pulmonary veins

Pulmonary artery

Bronchus

Pulmonary veins

ANTERIOR   **ANTERIOR**

B) Pulmonary arteries vs. bronchi

RALS

Right **A**nterior; **L**eft **S**uperior
In the **right lung**, the pulmonary arteries lie **anterior** to the bronchus, while in the **left lung** it lies **superior**.

128 Right vs. left bronchus

> **Inhaled objects go right down into the right bronchus**

The right bronchus is **shorter**, **wider**, and **more vertical** than the left, hence the majority of aspirated foreign bodies go down the right bronchus.

While upright: aspirated bodies usually enter the basal segments of the right lower lobe.
While supine: usually enter posterior segment of right upper lobe.
• Think about gravity and both locations will make sense!

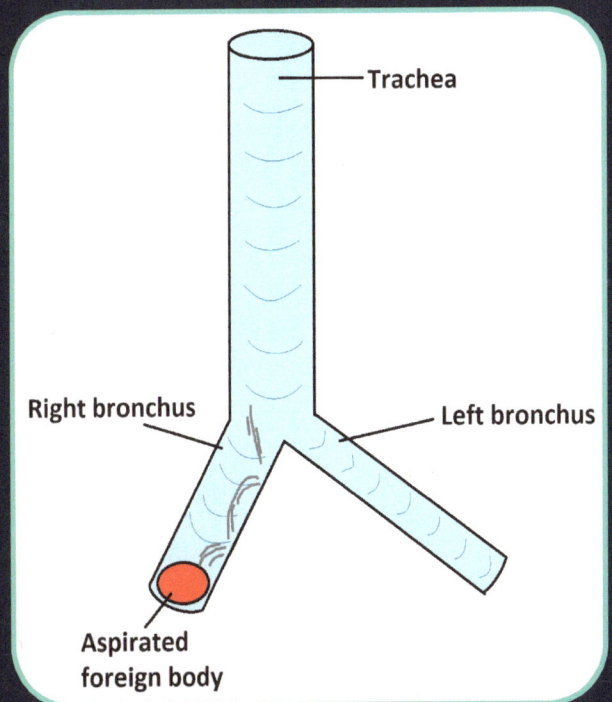

Trachea

Right bronchus

Left bronchus

Aspirated foreign body

129   Pharynx vs. larynx

> **Pharyx: Face**
> **Larynx: Lung pipe**

The **pharynx** is the part of the throat that lies at the level of the **face**. It extends down until the spot where it diverges into the larynx and esophagus.

The **larynx** ("voice box") is the start of the tract that goes to the **lungs**. It is located right below the pharynx.
- The **larynx** is responsible for **language/loudness** (i.e. it houses vocal cords, and manipulates pitch and volume)

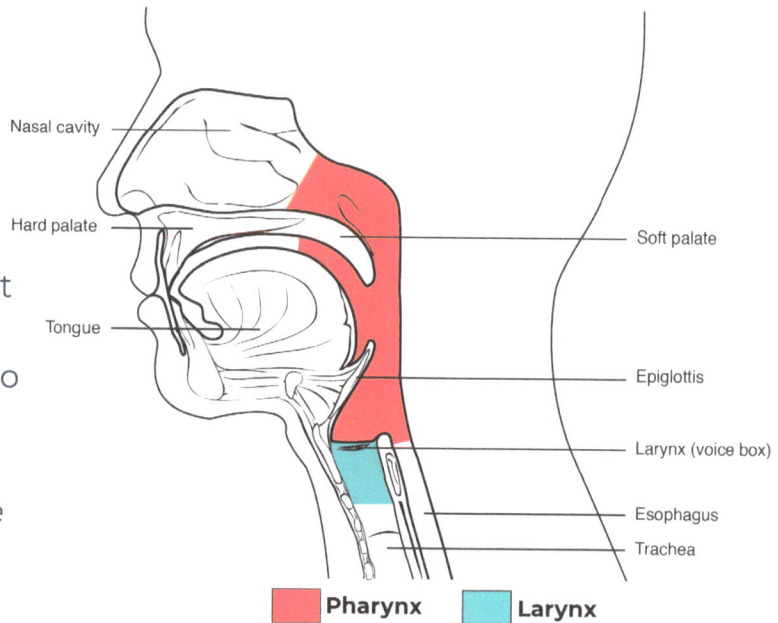

Labels: Nasal cavity, Hard palate, Tongue, Soft palate, Epiglottis, Larynx (voice box), Esophagus, Trachea

Pharynx   Larynx

130   Nasal turbinates (conchae)

> **Think of a wind turbine**

Nasal turbinates are narrow, curled ridges of bone that protrude into the breathing passage of the nose. They channel inhaled air into a steady, regular airflow, bearing resemblance to a **wind turbine** (hence the name '**turbinate**'). They also warm and moisten the inhaled air.

Simply think of a wind turbine and the location and function of nasal turbinates will become apparent!

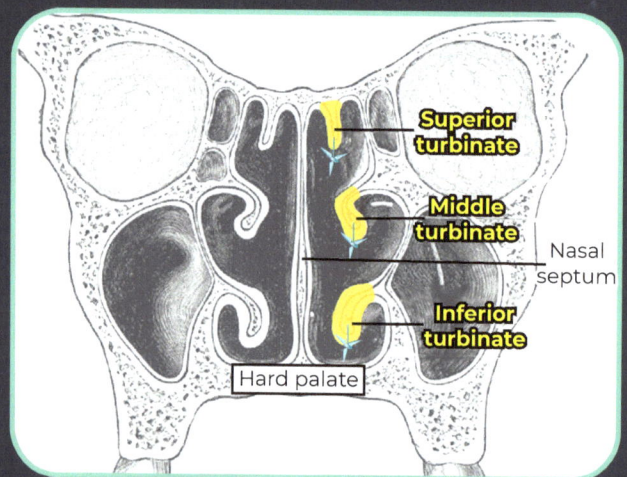

Labels: Superior turbinate, Middle turbinate, Inferior turbinate, Nasal septum, Hard palate

(!) When the turbinates get enlarged, for example due to allergies, they can cause **nasal obstruction**.

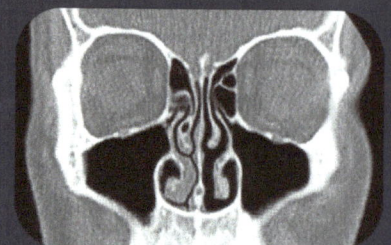

Right turbinates enlarged; left normal.

CHAPTER 14

Renal

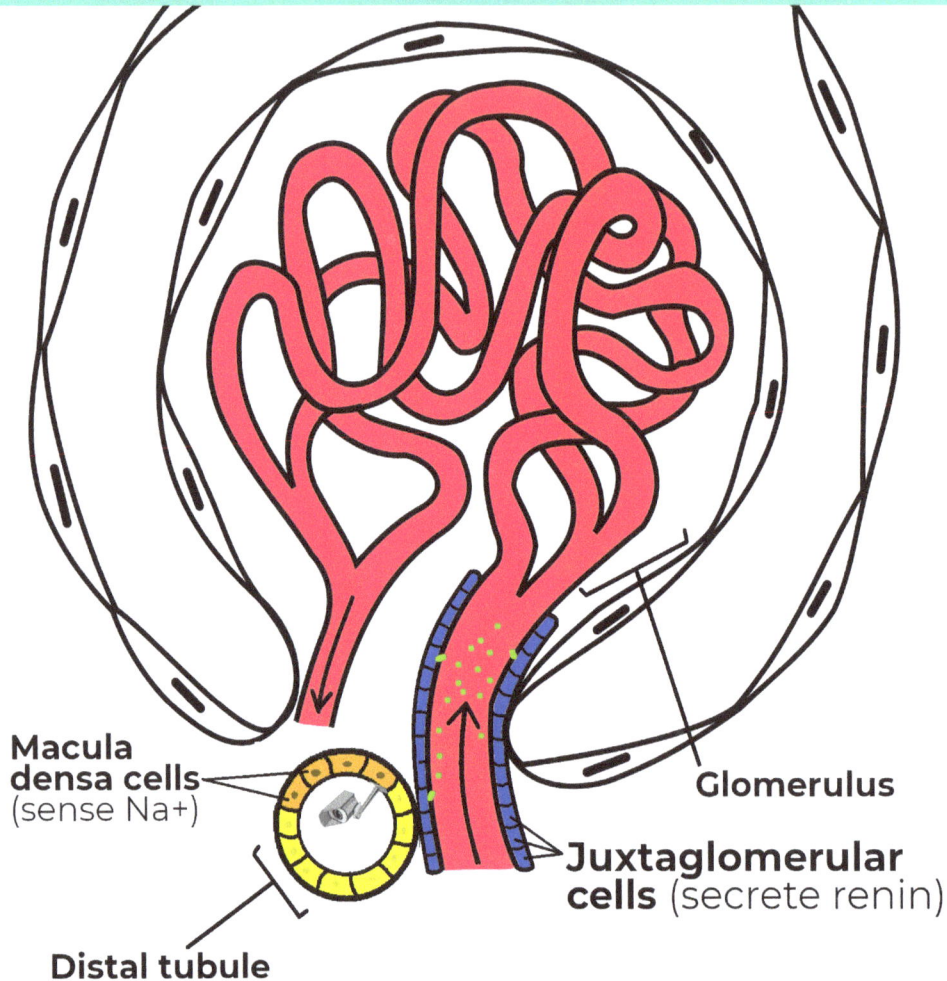

Macula densa cells (sense Na+)

Glomerulus

Juxtaglomerular cells (secrete renin)

Distal tubule

131 Juxtaglomerular apparatus

> Macula **densa**: salt *sensa*
> **Juxtaglomerular** cells: **juxtaposed** to the **glomerulus**

The juxtaglomerular apparatus functions to maintain glomerular filtration rate (GFR) via the renin-angiotensin-aldosterone system. It consists of 3 things:

1. Juxtaglomerular (JG) cells
- As implied by the name, these cells are **juxtaposed** (beside) to the **glomerulus** (specifically, they are smooth muscle of the **afferent arteriole**). It thus makes sense that they function to **secrete renin directly into the blood**.

2. Macula densa
- These cells are **NaCl sensors** located on the **distal tubule**. When they sense low NaCl, they signal to the JG cells to increase renin secretion.

3. Mesangial cells
- These are involved in mechanical roles/debris removal, and are generally not tested on very much.

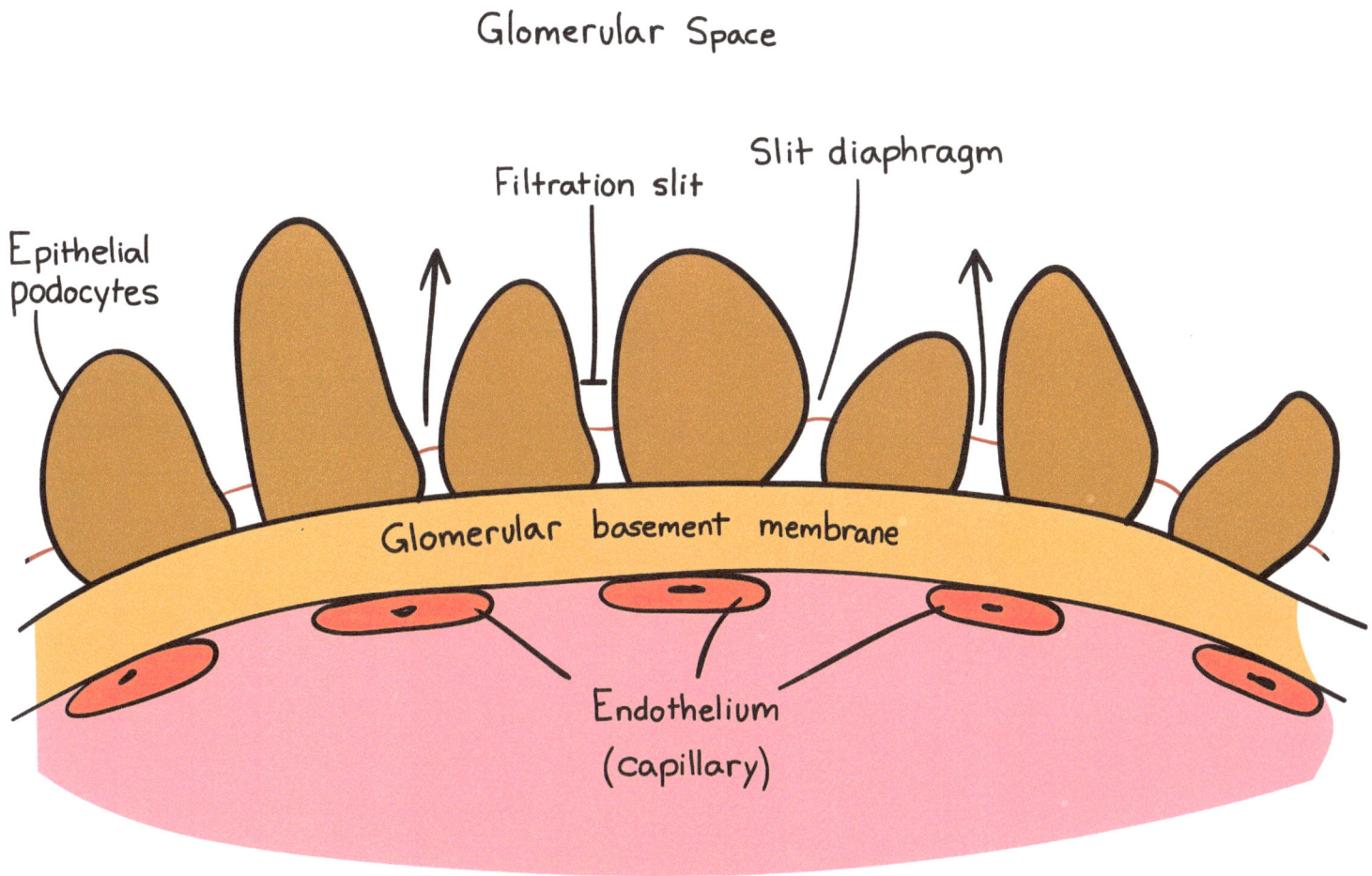

Glomerular Space

Filtration slit

Slit diaphragm

Epithelial
podocytes

Glomerular basement membrane

Endothelium
(capillary)

132 Glomerular filtration barrier

A **basement** between two **"-thelium"**s

The glomerular filtration barrier consists of 3 layers:
1. **Podocytes (epithelium)**
2. **Basement membrane**
3. **Endothelium (blood vessel)**

All 3 layers are **negatively charged**, which prevents passage of other negatively charged molecules, like albumin.

To remember the negative charge all 3 layers have, just look at the endothelium - it looks like a series of 'negative' signs.

- -

119

NOTES

CHAPTER 15

Reproductive

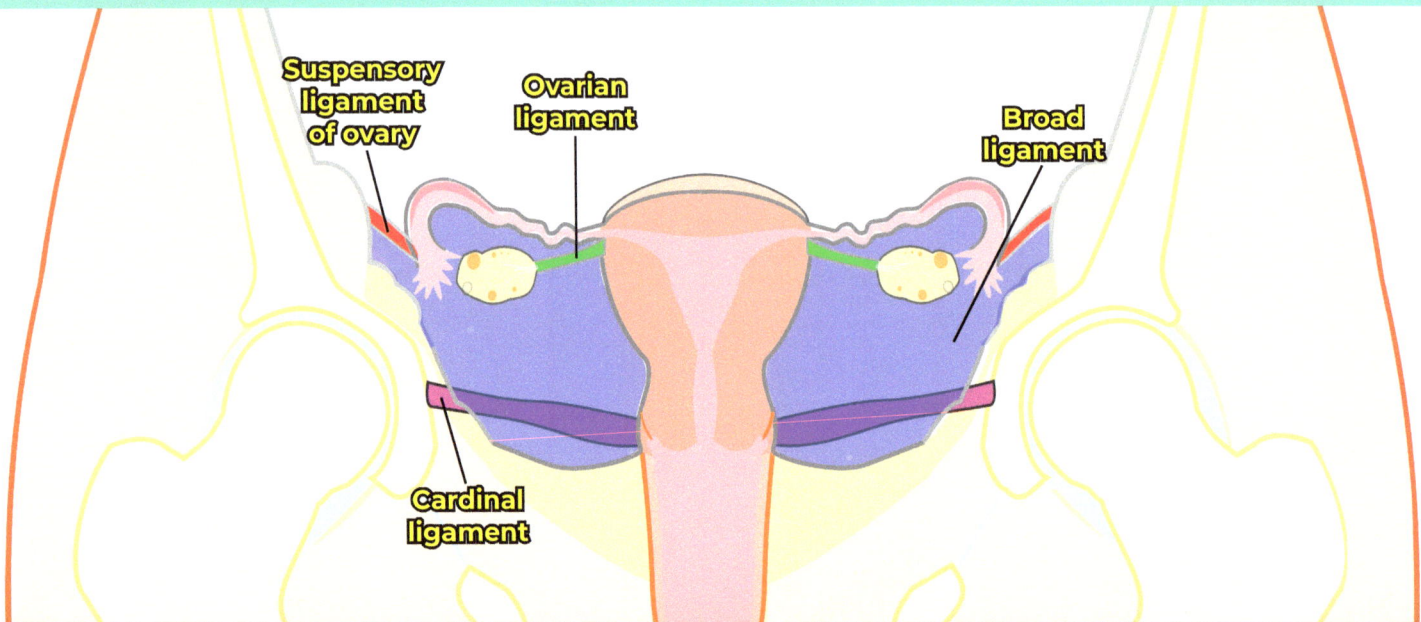

Suspensory ligament of ovary

Ovarian ligament

Broad ligament

Cardinal ligament

133 Female reproductive ligaments

IN THE NAME!

In the name

1. **Cardinal ligament**
   - Contains the **uterine vessels**
   - "Cardinal" means "**of the greatest importance**" - a befitting name, considering it contains the very important uterine vessels.
2. **Suspensory ligament of the ovary** (infundibulopelvic ligament)
   - Contains the **ovarian vessels**
   - The word "suspensory" hints that it must **come from above** to hold the ovary up. It thus makes sense that it contains the ovarian vessels, which originate SUPERIORLY from the aorta and IVC.
3. **Broad ligament**
   - Contains ovaries, fallopian tubes, and round ligament of uterus
   - Structurally ties the uterus, fallopian tubes, and ovaries to the pelvic side wall
   - The word "broad" literally tells you it is **broad** in size and in the structures it contains
4. **Ovarian ligament**
   - Connects the **ovary** to the uterus
5. **Round ligament of the uterus** (not shown)
   - Literally keeps the uterus **round** (maintains anteflexion and anteversion)
   - Travels through the *round* inguinal canal.

(!) **Round ligament pain:** When the uterus grows during pregnancy, it can stretch the round ligaments, causing pain. It is one of the most common discomforts of pregnancy.

134 Most common site of fertilization

Pregnancy gets amped up in the ampulla.

The most common site of fertilization is the **ampulla** of the fallopian tube. The fertilized egg then moves down the fallopian tube to implant into the endometrium of the uterus. If this migration doesn't happen, it results in an **ectopic pregnancy**.

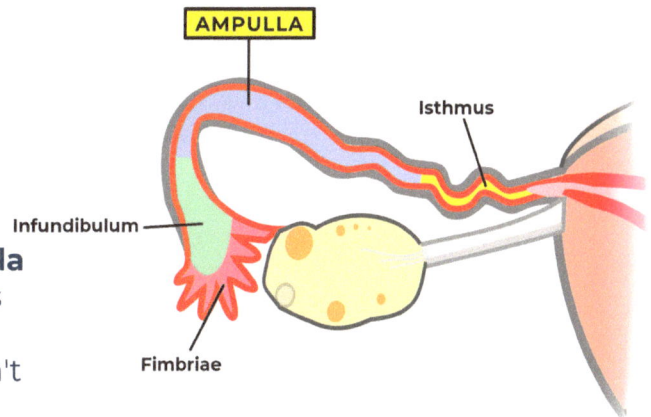

AMPULLA

Isthmus

Infundibulum

Fimbriae

135 Innervation of the male sexual response

"Point and Shoot!"

Erection: parasympathetic (pelvic nerve)
Ejaculation: somatic (pudendal nerve)

In addition to this mnemonic, the innervations can easily remembered using logic: generally for an erection to happen, the individual must be in a **relaxed (i.e. parasympathetic) state**. Ejaculation, on the other hand, is simply a **series of muscle contractions** rather than an arousal state - hence its innervation is via **somatic** (meaning *skeletal muscle*) nerves.

136 Layers of the scrotum

"Some Dang Englishman Called It The Testis!"

Layers of the scrotum (superficial to deep):

Skin
Dartos fascia
External spermatic fascia
Cremaster muscle
Internal spermatic fascia
Tunica vaginalis
Testis

Cremasteric reflex: stroking the inner thigh causes rise of the ipsilateral testicle due to cremasteric muscle contraction. It's almost always absent/diminished in **testicular torsion** (twisting of spermatic cord which cuts off blood flow). This makes sense - without sufficient blood flow, the muscle can't contract.

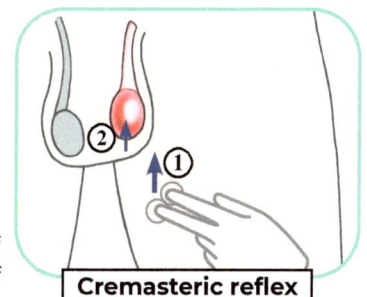

Cremasteric reflex

Tip: Just like the abdominal wall, the scrotum has a **muscle sandwich** - the cremasteric muscle, sandwiched between the external and internal spermatic fascia. Remember: fascia functions to keep muscles in place, hence it makes sense that there is fascia immediately above and below the cremasteric muscle.

NOTES

CREDITS

1. Human brainstem-thalamus posterior view description: (https://commons.wikimedia.org/wiki/File:Human_brainstem-thalamus_posterior_view_description.JPG) by John A Beal, PhD under CC BY 2.5 (https://creativecommons.org/licenses/by/2.5/deed.en)

2. Inferior colliculus - sagittal cut: (https://commons.wikimedia.org/wiki/File:Inferior_colliculus_-_sagittal_cut.jpg) by Graziano M (2014) How Ventriloquism Works under CC BY 3.0 (https://creativecommons.org/licenses/by/3.0/deed.en)

3. Image derivative of Liver 04 Couinaud classification: (https://commons.wikimedia.org/wiki/File:Liver_04_Couinaud_classification.svg) by Database Center for Life Science under CC BY-SA 2.1 JP (https://creativecommons.org/licenses/by-sa/2.1/jp/deed.en)

4. Left atrial enlargement radiograph courtesy of Dr Ahmed Abdrabou, <ahref="https://radiopaedia.org/">Radiopaedia.org</a>. From the case <ahref="https://radiopaedia.org/cases/23098">rID: 23098</a>

5. Image derivative of Hypophyse: (https://commons.wikimedia.org/wiki/File:Hypophyse.png) by Patrick J. Lynch under CC BYSA 3.0 (https://creativecommons.org/licenses/by-sa/3.0/deed.en)

6. Image derivative of 3D Medical Animation Spleen Anatomy: (https://commons.wikimedia.org/wiki/File:3D_Medical_Animation_Spleen_Anatomy.jpg) by https://www.scienti_canimations.com under CC BY-SA 4.0 (https://creativecommons.org/licenses/by-sa/4.0/deed.en)

7. Image derivative of BodyParts3D Rib cage: (https://commons.wikimedia.org/wiki/File:BodyParts3D_Rib_cage.stl) by BodyParts3D under CC BY-SA 2.1 JP (https://creativecommons.org/licenses/by-sa/2.1/jp/deed.en)

8. Glomerular filtration barrier image by Khan Academy: (https://www.khanacademy.org/test-prep/mcat/organ-systems/the-renal-system/a/renalphysiology-glomerular-filtration) under CC BY-NC-SA 4.0 (https://creativecommons.org/licenses/by-nc-sa/4.0/)

9. Image derivative of Scheme female reproductive non-labels: (https://commons.wikimedia.org/wiki/File:Scheme_female_reproductive_non-labels.svg) by Jmarchn under CC BY-SA 3.0 (https://creativecommons.org/licenses/by-sa/3.0/deed.en)

10. Image derivative of Brain human normal inferior view with labels en-2: (https://commons.wikimedia.org/wiki/File:Brain_human_normal_inferior_view_with_labels_en-2.svg) by Patrick J. Lynch under CC BY 2.5 (https://creativecommons.org/licenses/by/2.5/deed.en)

11. Image derivative of Meninges-en: (https://commons.wikimedia.org/wiki/File:Meningesen.svg) by SEER Development Team under CC BY-SA 3.0 (https://creativecommons.org/licenses/by-sa/3.0/deed.en)

12. Syringomyelia (with arrow) image: (https://commons.wikimedia.org/wiki/File:Syringomyelia_(with_arrow).png) by Cyborg Ninja at English Wikipedia under CC BY 4.0 (https://creativecommons.org/licenses/by/4.0/deed.en)

13. Unilateral hypoglossal nerve injury image: (https://commons.wikimedia.org/wiki/File:Unilateral_hypoglossal_nerve_injury.jpeg) by Mukherjee SK, Gowshami CB, Salam A, Kuddus R, Farazi MA, Baksh J under CC BY 2.0 (https://creativecommons.org/licenses/by/2.0/deed.en)

14. Image derivative of Diagram showing the lining of the lungs (the pleura) CRUK 306: (https://commons.wikimedia.org/wikiFile:Diagram_showing_the_lining_of_the_lungs_(the_pleura)_CRUK_306.svg) by Cancer Research UK under CC BY-SA 4.0 (https://creativecommons.org/licenses/by-sa/4.0/deed.en)

15. Image derivative of Scapula Winging in Long Thoracic Nerve Palsy: (https://commons.wikimedia.org/wiki/File:Scapula_Winging_in_Long_Thoracic_Nerve_Palsy.jpg) by Dwaipayanc under CC BY-SA 3.0: (https://creativecommons.org/licenses/bysa/3.0/deed.en)

16. Image derivative of Tractus intestinalis rectum: (https://commons.wikimedia.org/wiki/File:Tractus_intestinalis_rectum.svg) by Olek Remesz under CC BY-SA 2.5 (https://creativecommons.org/licenses/by-sa/2.5/deed.en)

17. Free Nerve Endings: (https://commons.wikimedia.org/wiki/File:Blausen_0803_Skin_FreeNerveEndings.png) by Bruce Blaus under CC BY 3.0 (https://creativecommons.org/licenses/by/3.0/deed.en)

18. Intrinsic muscles of the foot: (https://commons.wikimedia.org/wiki/File:1124_Intrinsic_Muscles_of_the_Foot_b.png) by OpenStax College under CC BY 3.0 (https://creativecommons.org/licenses/by/3.0/deed.en)

19. Side Views of the Muscles of Facial Expression Numbered: (https://commons.wikimedia.org/wiki/File:1106_Side_Views_of_the_Muscles_of_Facial_Expressions_numbered.jpg) by CNX Anatomy 2013 under CC BY 4.0 (https://creativecommons.org/licenses/by/4.0/deed.en)

20. Left Lateral Malleolus Avulsion Fracture: (https://commons.wikimedia.org/wiki/File:Left_lateral_malleolus_avulsion_fracture.jpg) by Tim D Williamson under CC BY-SA 4.0 (https://creativecommons.org/licenses/by-sa/4.0/deed.en)

21. Tib fib growth plates: (https://commons.wikimedia.org/wiki/File:Tib_fib_growth_plates.jpg) by Gilo1969 under CC BY 3.0 (https://creativecommons.org/licenses/by/3.0/deed.en)

22. Organe-brust-bauch: (https://commons.wikimedia.org/wiki/File:Organe-brust-bauch-br03.jpg) by Beat Ruest under CC BY-SA 4.0 (https://creativecommons.org/licenses/by-sa/4.0/deed.en)

23. 1121 Intrinsic Muscles of the Hand PIL: (https://commons.wikimedia.org/wiki/File:1121_Intrinsic_Muscles_of_the_Hand_PIL.png) by CFCF under CC BY-SA 4.0 (https://creativecommons.org/licenses/by-sa/4.0/deed.en)

24. DRG Chicken e7: (https://commons.wikimedia.org/wiki/File:DRG_Chicken_e7.jpg) by Dp under CC BY-SA 2.5 (https://creativecommons.org/licenses/by-sa/2.5/deed.en)

25. Figure 35 04 04: (https://commons.wikimedia.org/wiki/File:Figure_35_04_04.jpg) by CNX OpenStax under CC BY 4.0 (https://creativecommons.org/licenses/by/4.0/deed.en)

26. Human brain right dissected lateral view description: (https://commons.wikimedia.org/wiki/File:Human_brain_right_dissected_lateral_view_description.JPG) by John A Beal, PhD under CC BY 2.5 (https://creativecommons.org/licenses/by/2.5/deed.en)

27. Lissencephaly: (https://commons.wikimedia.org/wiki/File:Lissencephaly.jpg) by Lefèvre J, Mangin J-F (2010) under CC BY 2.5 (https://creativecommons.org/licenses/by/2.5/deed.en)

28. Anatomical snuff box2: (https://commons.wikimedia.org/wiki/File:Anatomical_snuff_box2.jpg) by Enterim under CC BY-SA 4.0 (https://creativecommons.org/licenses/by-sa/4.0/deed.en)

29. Leg compartments: (https://commons.wikimedia.org/wiki/File:Leg_compartments.jpg) by Khan IA, Mahabadi N, D'Abarno A, et al. (2019) under CC BY 4.0 (https://creativecommons.org/licenses/by/4.0/deed.en)

30. Chordae tendinae papillary muscles: (https://commons.wikimedia.org/wiki/File:2010_Chordae_Tendinae_Papillary_Muscles.jpg) by OpenStax College under CC BY 3.0 (https://creativecommons.org/licenses/by/3.0/deed.en)

31. Pneumothorax: (https://commons.wikimedia.org/wiki/File:Blausen_0742_Pneumothorax.png) by BruceBlaus under CC BY 3.0 (https://creativecommons.org/licenses/by/3.0/deed.en)

32. Cardiac tamponade: (https://commons.wikimedia.org/wiki/File:Blausen_0164_CardiacTamponade_02.png) by BruceBlaus under CC BY 3.0 (https://creativecommons.org/licenses/by/3.0/deed.en)

33. Pectoralis minor: (https://commons.wikimedia.org/wiki/File:Pectoralis_minor.svg) by Användare:Chrizz under CC BY-SA 3.0 (https://creativecommons.org/licenses/by-sa/3.0/deed.en)

34. Fibularis longus and fibularis brevis: (https://en.wikipedia.org/wiki/File:Lateral_compartment_of_leg_-_Fibularis_longus.png and https://commons.wikimedia.org/wiki/File:Lateral_compartment_of_leg_-_Fibularis_brevis.png) by BodyParts3D under CC-BY-SA 2.1 JP (https://creativecommons.org/licenses/by-sa/2.1/jp/deed.en)

35. Planes of body: (https://commons.wikimedia.org/wiki/File:Planes_of_Body.jpg) by OpenStax College under CC BY 3.0 (https://creativecommons.org/licenses/by/3.0/deed.en)

36. Body movements I: (https://commons.wikimedia.org/wiki/File:Body_Movements_I.jpg) by Tonye Ogele CNX under CC BY-SA 3.0 (https://creativecommons.org/licenses/by-sa/3.0/deed.en)

37. Biceps brachii muscle: and triceps brachii muscle: (https://commons.wikimedia.org/wiki/File:Biceps_brachii_muscle06.png and https://commons.wikimedia.org/wiki/File:Triceps_brachii_muscle10.png) by Anatomography under CC BY-SA 2.1 (https://creativecommons.org/licenses/by-sa/2.1/jp/deed.en)

38. DoubleJ: (https://commons.wikimedia.org/wiki/File:DoubleJ.jpg) by Lucien Monfils under CC BY-SA 3.0 (https://creativecommons.org/licenses/by-sa/3.0/deed.en)

39. Voluculus: (https://commons.wikimedia.org/wiki/File:Voluculus.PNG) by James Heilman, MD under CC BY-SA 3.0 (https://creativecommons.org/licenses/by-sa/3.0/deed.en)

40. Cranial fossae: (https://commons.wikimedia.org/wiki/File:Cranial_fossae_boundaries.svg) by BodyParts3D under CC BY-SA 2.1 JP (https://creativecommons.org/licenses/by-sa/2.1/jp/deed.en)

41. Iliac fossa: (https://commons.wikimedia.org/wiki/File:Iliac_fossa_02_anterior_view.png) by BodyParts3D under CC BY-SA 2.1 JP (https://creativecommons.org/licenses/by-sa/2.1/jp/deed.en)

42. Brachial plexus: (https://commons.wikimedia.org/wiki/File:Brachial_plexus_.jpg) by Alice Roberts under CC BY 2.0 (https://creativecommons.org/licenses/by/2.0/deed.en)

43. Ruptured achilles tendon (https://commons.wikimedia.org/wiki/File:Rupture_tendon_achil%C3%A9en.jpg) by Grook Da Oger under CC BY-SA 3.0 (https://creativecommons.org/licenses/by-sa/3.0/deed.en)

44. Arteries of the brain: (https://commons.wikimedia.org/wiki/File:2123_Arteries_of_the_Brain.jpg) by OpenStax College under CC BY 3.0 (https://creativecommons.org/licenses/by/3.0/deed.en)

45. Types of neuroglia: (https://commons.wikimedia.org/wiki/File:Blausen_0870_TypesofNeuroglia.png#/media/File:Blausen_0870_TypesofNeuroglia.png) by BruceBlaus under CC BY 3.0 (https://creativecommons.org/licenses/by/3.0/deed.en)

46. Knee injury: (https://commons.wikimedia.org/wiki/File:918_Knee_Injury.jpg) by OpenStax College under CC BY 3.0 (https://creativecommons.org/licenses/by/3.0/deed.en)

47. Hem1 Basophile: (https://commons.wikimedia.org/wiki/File:Hem1Basophile.jpg) by El*Falaf under CC BY 3.0 (https://creativecommons.org/licenses/by/3.0/deed.en)

48. Eosinophil: (https://pixnio.com/science/microscopy-images/malaria-plasmodium/the-gametocytes-are-infectious-when-ingested-in-the-intestine-of-the-mosquito) by Dr. Mae Melvin, USCDCP under CC BY 3.0 (https://creativecommons.org/licenses/by/3.0/deed.en)

49. Neutrophil in a Blood Smear: (https://commons.wikimedia.org/wiki/File:Neutrophil_in_a_blood_smear.jpg) by hematologist under CC BY 3.0 (https://creativecommons.org/licenses/by/3.0/deed.en)

www.ingramcontent.com/pod-product-compliance
Lightning Source LLC
Chambersburg PA
CBHW050908210326
41597CB00002B/62